Ewa Meyer-Blazejewska

Stem cell-based therapy of ocular surface diseases

Ewa Meyer-Blazejewska

Stem cell-based therapy of ocular surface diseases

Novel approaches to expansion of adult epithelial stem cells in culture

Südwestdeutscher Verlag für Hochschulschriften

Impressum/Imprint (nur für Deutschland/ only for Germany)
Bibliografische Information der Deutschen Nationalbibliothek: Die Deutsche Nationalbibliothek verzeichnet diese Publikation in der Deutschen Nationalbibliografie; detaillierte bibliografische Daten sind im Internet über http://dnb.d-nb.de abrufbar.

Alle in diesem Buch genannten Marken und Produktnamen unterliegen warenzeichen-, marken- oder patentrechtlichem Schutz bzw. sind Warenzeichen oder eingetragene Warenzeichen der jeweiligen Inhaber. Die Wiedergabe von Marken, Produktnamen, Gebrauchsnamen, Handelsnamen, Warenbezeichnungen u.s.w. in diesem Werk berechtigt auch ohne besondere Kennzeichnung nicht zu der Annahme, dass solche Namen im Sinne der Warenzeichen- und Markenschutzgesetzgebung als frei zu betrachten wären und daher von jedermann benutzt werden dürften.

Verlag: Südwestdeutscher Verlag für Hochschulschriften Aktiengesellschaft & Co. KG
Dudweiler Landstr. 99, 66123 Saarbrücken, Deutschland
Telefon +49 681 37 20 271-1, Telefax +49 681 37 20 271-0
Email: info@svh-verlag.de
Zugl.: Erlangen, Friedrich-Alexander-Universität, Diss., 2009

Herstellung in Deutschland:
Schaltungsdienst Lange o.H.G., Berlin
Books on Demand GmbH, Norderstedt
Reha GmbH, Saarbrücken
Amazon Distribution GmbH, Leipzig
ISBN: 978-3-8381-1387-6

Imprint (only for USA, GB)
Bibliographic information published by the Deutsche Nationalbibliothek: The Deutsche Nationalbibliothek lists this publication in the Deutsche Nationalbibliografie; detailed bibliographic data are available in the Internet at http://dnb.d-nb.de.

Any brand names and product names mentioned in this book are subject to trademark, brand or patent protection and are trademarks or registered trademarks of their respective holders. The use of brand names, product names, common names, trade names, product descriptions etc. even without a particular marking in this works is in no way to be construed to mean that such names may be regarded as unrestricted in respect of trademark and brand protection legislation and could thus be used by anyone.

Publisher: Südwestdeutscher Verlag für Hochschulschriften Aktiengesellschaft & Co. KG
Dudweiler Landstr. 99, 66123 Saarbrücken, Germany
Phone +49 681 37 20 271-1, Fax +49 681 37 20 271-0
Email: info@svh-verlag.de

Printed in the U.S.A.
Printed in the U.K. by (see last page)
ISBN: 978-3-8381-1387-6

Copyright © 2010 by the author and Südwestdeutscher Verlag für Hochschulschriften Aktiengesellschaft & Co. KG and licensors
All rights reserved. Saarbrücken 2010

Index

1. **ABSTRACT** 3
    1.1. ABSTRACT ENGLISH 3
    1.2. ZUSAMMENFASSUNG DEUTSCH 5
2. **INTRODUCTION** 8
    2.1. CORNEAL EPITHELIAL CELLS AND THEIR NICHE 8
    2.2. CURRENT THERAPIES FOR UNILATERAL/BILATERAL LIMBAL STEM CELL DEFICIENCY 10
        2.2.1 Unilateral stem cell deficiency 11
        2.2.2. Bilateral stem cell deficiency 11
    2.3. OBJECTIVES: OPTIMIZATION OF CULTURE CONDITIONS AND SEARCH FOR ALTERNATIVE AUTOLOGOUS STEM CELL SOURCES 12
3. **MATERIALS AND METHODS** 14
    3.1. ANIMALS, TISSUES AND CELL LINES 14
        3.1.1. Animals 14
        3.1.2. Tissues 14
        3.1.3. Cell lines 14
    3.2. CHEMICALS AND EXPENDABLE MATERIALS 15
        3.2.1. Chemicals 15
        3.2.2. Enzymes 16
        3.2.3. Culture media and wares 16
        3.2.4. Growth factors 17
        3.2.5. Antibodies 17
        3.2.6. Primers 19
        3.2.7. Kits 20
        3.2.8. Surgical instruments 20
    3.3. EQUIPMENT AND SOFTWARE 20
        3.3.1. Equipment 20
        3.3.2. Software 21
    3.4. CELL CULTURE 21
        3.4.1. Dissociation and separation methods 21
        3.4.1.1. Fluorescence-activated cell sorting 22
        3.4.2. Cell culture under various culture conditions 22
        3.4.3. Clonal expansion on a 3T3 feeder cell layer 23
    3.5. CLONAL GROWTH ASSAY 24
    3.6. COATING OF CHAMBER SLIDES WITH EXTRACELLULAR MATRIX COMPONENTS 24
    3.7. CONDITIONING OF CULTURE MEDIUM WITH CORNEAL AND LIMBAL EPITHELIAL CELLS AND STROMAL FIBROBLASTS 24
    3.8. SUBCULTURE OF CLONAL CELLS UNDER VARIOUS ENVIRONMENTAL CONDITIONS 25
    3.9. GENERATION OF EPITHELIAL SHEETS ON FIBRIN 25
    3.10. METHODS OF EVALUATION 26
        3.10.1. Light and electron microscopy 26

    3.10.2. Immunohisto-/cytochemistry..26
    3.10.3. Real-Time RT-PCR...27
    3.10.4. Western Blot Analysis 27
  3.11. ENGRAFTMENT OF CULTIVATED HAIR FOLLICLE EPITHELIAL SHEETS 28
  3.12. STATISTICS...28

4. RESULTS..29

  4.1. OPTIMIZATION OF CULTURE CONDITIONS FOR EXPANSION OF LIMBAL STEM AND PROGENITOR CELLS 29
    4.1.1. Clonal growth and phenotypic characterization...29
    4.1.2. Effect of limbal region and donor age on clonal growth..32
    4.1.3. Effect of dissociation method on clonal growth 34
    4.1.4. Effect of culture conditions on clonal growth..34
    4.1.5. Effect of culture conditions on clonal cell phenotype 38
    4.1.6. Generation of epithelial cell sheets on fibrin..40
  4.2. ALTERNATIVE AUTOLOGOUS STEM CELL SOURCES: MURINE AND HUMAN HAIR FOLLICLES 42
    4.2.1. Comparative expression of stem cell and differentiation markers in hair follicles and cornea. 42
    4.2.2. Isolation and clonal enrichment of murine and human hair follicle bulge cells........................43
    4.2.3. Effect of environmental conditions on growth and differentiation of murine and human hair follicle stem cells 48
    4.2.4. Premilinary engraftment experiments of cultivated hair follicle epithelial sheets 55

5. DISCUSSION 58

  5.1. OPTIMIZATION OF CELL CULTURE CONDITIONS FOR EX VIVO EXPANSION OF LIMBAL EPITHELIAL STEM AND PROGENITOR CELLS 58
  5.2. ALTERNATIVE SOURCES OF ADULT EPITHELIAL STEM CELLS: TRANSDIFFERENTIATION OF MURINE AND HUMAN HAIR FOLLICLE 61
  5.3 CONCLUSIONS 63

6. REFERENCES 65

7. ABBREVIATIONS 73

1. Abstract

1.1. Abstract English

Homeostasis of corneal epithelial cells is an important prerequisite not only for the integrity of the ocular surface but also for corneal transparency and visual function. The continuous renewal of the corneal epithelium is provided by a population of stem cells (SC) located in the basal epithelium of the limbus, a transitional zone between the corneal and the neighbouring conjunctival epithelium. In cases of a partial or total depletion of limbal epithelial SC, termed limbal SC deficiency, the conjunctival epithelium migrates over the surface of the cornea causing vascularisation, recurrent epithelial erosion, and chronic inflammation leading to severe visual impairment and ultimately blindness.

One emerging surgical strategy for restoring a normal corneal epithelial surface in patients with limbal SC deficiency is transplantation of *ex vivo* expanded limbal epithelial SC which represents one of the few adult human SC therapies being currently employed. In unilaterally affected patients, this therapeutic approach commonly involves the harvest of a small limbal biopsy from the patient´s contralateral healthy eye followed by cell expansion *ex vivo* to generate an epithelial sheet on a transplantable carrier such as amniotic membrane or fibrin gel. Although successful restoration of the ocular surface occurs in the early postoperative period, the long-term outcome is less satisfactory, most probably due to depletion of limbal SC in culture. In patients with bilateral limbal SC deficiency, cadaveric donor eyes or alternative autologous SC sources such as oral mucosa or conjunctiva are required which, however, have provided less satisfactory long-term clinical outcomes so far. Therefore, present research activities focus on the evaluation of further alternative autologous SC sources for *ex vivo* culture and transplantation avoiding the risk of immune-mediated rejection or the need for immunosuppression.

Since the long-term clinical outcome of the currently employed limbal SC therapies has not yet been proved satisfactory, the major objective of this work was, in general, to establish novel SC-based cultivation techniques for therapeutic applications in patients with unilateral or bilateral limbal SC deficiency. In particular, the purpose of this study was (1) to provide an optimized culture method supporting the preferential expansion and maintenance of limbal SC throughout the cultivation process, and (2) to explore the suitability of hair follicle (HF) as an alternative autologous SC source and the potential of HF-derived SC to transdifferentiate into corneal epithelial-like cells when exposed to a specific microenvironment.

In order to provide an optimized culture protocol for limbal SC, the effect of several culture variables, such as limbal biopsy regions, dissociation methods, culture media as well as calcium, serum and growth factor concentrations, on clonal growth and differentiation of limbal SC was systematically analysed. Maintenance of SC phenotype within the cultivated epithelial cell sheets

Abstract

was evaluated by means of morphological and immunohistochemical methods using antibodies against established SC markers. In order to investigate the capacity of HF epithelial SC to transdifferentiate into a corneal epithelial-like phenotype, HF-derived SC were exposed to cornea- or limbus-specific microenvironmental factors, such as specific extracellular matrix components or soluble growth and survival factors contained within conditioned media of tissue-specific fibroblasts. Cellular phenotype and differentiation of cultured cell sheets were evaluated by means of histological, molecular and immunohistochemical methods using antibodies against SC and tissue-specific differentiation markers.

Clonal analysis showed that limbal cells obtained from the superior limbus, isolated by a gentle two-step enzymatic dissociation method (dispase II/trypsin-EDTA), cultured in low to medium (0.03-0.4 mmol/l) calcium concentrations with proper serum levels (10%) and growth factor combinations (EGF/NGF) yielded the highest clonal growth capacity and an undifferentiated cellular phenotype. Subsequent subcultivation of clonal cells on fibrin gels supported the preservation of stem and progenitor cells within the transplantable epithelial cell sheets as demonstrated by multiple molecular SC markers. The transdifferentiation experiments showed that both murine and human HF-derived epithelial SC could be induced to transdifferentiate into a corneal-epithelial-like phenotype, when exposed to a limbus-specific microenvironment, i.e. laminin-5 as substrate and conditioned medium from limbal stromal fibroblasts. These limbal niche factors significantly upregulated expression of cornea-specific K12- and Pax6- mRNA and protein, whereas expression of the epidermal keratinocyte marker K10 was significantly downregulated.

These findings indicate, that using clonal expansion, subcultivation of clonal cells on fibrin gels, and specific culture methods, which support enrichment and preservation of the SC phenotype during the entire cultivation process, multilayered transplantable sheets of epithelial cells can be generated from small human limbal biopsy specimens. This proposed culture system may be essential for long-term clinical success and wide-spread use of this SC-based therapy and may contribute to restoration of the ocular surface in patients with unilateral limbal SC deficiency. Furthermore, HF may be an easily accessible alternative source of autologous adult SC and a promising therapeutic tool for replacement of the corneal epithelium and restoration of visual function in patients with bilateral ocular surface disorders.

1.2. Zusammenfassung Deutsch

Die Homöostase des Hornhautepithels ist eine grundlegende Voraussetzung nicht nur für die Integrität der Augenoberfläche, sondern auch für die Transparenz der Hornhaut und das Sehvermögen. Die stetige Erneuerung des Hornhautepithels wird durch eine Population von Stammzellen, die in der basalen Epithelschicht des Limbus, der Übergangsregion zwischen Hornhaut und Bindehaut, lokalisiert ist, gewährleistet. Bei teilweiser oder vollständiger Disfunktion dieser Stammzellen, der sog. Limbusstammzellinsuffizienz, wächst das benachbarte Bindehautepithel über die Hornhautoberfläche und führt zu Vaskularisierung, rezidivierenden epithelialen Erosionen und chronischer Entzündung, die zur Beeinträchtigung des Sehvermögens bis hin zur Erblindung führen.

Eine der neueren operativen Strategien zur Wiederherstellung der gesunden Hornhautepitheloberfläche bei Patienten mit limbaler Stammzellinsuffizienz ist die Transplantation von *ex vivo* expandierten limbalen epithelialen Stammzellen, welche eine der wenigen derzeit verwendeten Therapieansätze mit Einsatz von adulten Stammzellen repräsentiert. Bei Patienten mit einseitiger limbaler Stammzellinsuffizienz umfasst dieser Therapieansatz normalerweise die Entnahme von kleinen limbalen Gewebebiopsien vom gesunden Partnerauge des Patienten, die Isolation und *ex vivo* - Expansion der epithelialen Stammzellen sowie die Kultivierung eines epithelialen Zellverbands auf transplantierbarem Trägermaterial, wie z.B. Fibringel oder Amnionmembran. Trotz erfolgreicher Rekonstruktion der Augenoberfläche in der frühen postoperativen Phase ist der Langzeiterfolg dieser Therapiestrategie bislang wenig zufrieden stellend. Bei Patienten mit bilateraler limbaler Stammzellinsuffizienz werden entweder Limbus-Gewebe von Spenderaugen oder andere autologe Stammzellquellen, wie z.B. Mundschleimhaut oder Bindehaut, benötigt, womit allerdings bisher wenig zufrieden stellende klinische Langzeitergebnisse erzielt werden konnten. Deshalb konzentrieren sich derzeitige Forschungsschwerpunkte auf die Evaluierung weiterer alternativer autologer Stammzellquellen zur Rekonstruktion und Transplantation von Hornhautepitheläquivalenten, um die Risiken einer immunologischen Abstoßung oder immunsuppressiven Therapie zu umgehen.

Da sich der klinische Langzeiterfolg der gegenwärtig angewandten limbalen Stammzelltherapien bisher nicht als zufrieden stellend erwiesen hat, war das Hauptziel dieser Arbeit im Allgemeinen, neue Stammzell-basierte Kultivierungstechniken für therapeutische Anwendungen an Patienten mit uni- oder bilateraler Stammzellinsuffizienz zu etablieren. Im Speziellen wurde zunächst versucht, eine optimierte Kultivierungsmethode für limbale Stammzellen zu entwickeln, die die spezifische Anreicherung und Erhaltung des Stammzellphänotyps während des gesamten Kultivierungsprozesses unterstützt. Desweiteren wurde untersucht, ob sich Haarfollikel als alternative Stammzellquelle eignen und ein

Zusammenfassung

Transdifferenzierungspotential für einen Hornhautepithel-ähnlichen Phänotyp besitzen, wenn sie dem Einfluss Hornhaut/Limbus- spezifischer exogener Faktoren ausgesetzt werden.

Um ein optimiertes Kultivierungsprotokoll für limbale Stammzellen zu etablieren, wurden die Effekte verschiedener Kulturvariablen, wie z.B. die Biopsatregion-Entnahme, Zellisolierungsmethoden, Kulturmedien sowie Kalzium-, Serum- und Wachstumsfaktor-Konzentrationen, auf klonales Wachstum und Differenzierung limbaler Stammzellen systematisch untersucht. Die Erhaltung des Stammzell-Phänotyps innerhalb der kultivierten epithelialen Zellschichten wurde mit Hilfe von morphologischen und immunhistochemischen Methoden unter Verwendung von Antikörpern gegen etablierte Stammzell-Marker analysiert. Um die Kapazität epithelialer Haarfollikel-Stammzellen, sich in einen Hornhautepithel-ähnlichen Phänotyp zu differenzieren, zu evaluieren, wurden diese Hornhaut- und Limbus-spezifischen exogenen Faktoren, wie z.B. spezifischen extrazellulären Matrixkomponenten oder in konditionierten Medien enthaltenen löslichen Faktoren, ausgesetzt. Zellulärer Phänotyp und Differenzierung der kultivierten Zellschichten wurden mit Hilfe von histologischen, molekularen und immunhistochemischen Methoden unter Verwendung von Antikörpern gegen Stammzell- und Gewebe-spezifische Marker evaluiert.

Klonale Analysen zeigten, dass die vom superioren Limbus gewonnenen Stammzellen, die mittels einer zweistufigen enzymatischen Dissoziationsmethode (Dispasell/Trypsin-EDTA) isoliert, und in Kulturmedium mit niedriger bis mittlerer Kalziumkonzentration (0,03 – 0,4 mmol/l), geeigneter Serumkonzentration (10%) und Wachstumsfaktorkombination (EGF/NGF) kultiviert wurden, die höchste klonale Wachstumskapazität und einen undifferenzierten Phänotyp aufwiesen. Die anschließende Subkultivierung der klonal angereicherten Zellen auf Fibringelen förderte die Erhaltung der Stamm- und Vorläuferzellen in den zu transplantierenden Zellschichten, was mit Hilfe zahlreicher molekularer Stammzellmarker nachgewiesen werden konnte. Die Transdifferenzierungsexperimente legten dar, dass sich sowohl murine als auch humane Haarfollikel Stammzellen in einen Hornhautepithel-ähnlichen Phänotyp differenzieren konnten, wenn sie limbus-spezifischen exogenen Faktoren, wie z.B. Laminin-5 als Substrat und konditioniertem Medium aus limbalen stromalen Fibroblasten, ausgesetzt wurden. Unter dem Einfluss dieser limbalen Nischenfaktoren stieg die Expression Hornhaut-spezifischer Marker, wie K12- und Pax6- mRNA und Protein, in den Haarfollikelzellen signifikant an, während die Expression epidermaler Keratinozyten-Marker, wie K10, signifikant herunterreguliert wurde.

Diese Ergebnisse belegen, dass mittels klonaler Expansion, Subkultivierung der klonal angereicherten Stammzellen auf Fibringelen und spezifischer Kultivierungsmethoden, die die Anreicherung und Erhaltung des Stammzell-Phänotyps während des gesamten Kultivierungsprozesses fördern, mehrschichtige transplantierbare Epithelzellschichten aus kleinen limbalen Biopsaten hergestellt werden können. Dieses entwickelte Kultivierungssystem könnte essentiell für einen langfristigen klinischen Erfolg und eine weit verbreitete Anwendung dieser Stammzell-basierten Therapiestrategie sein und zur dauerhaften Wiederherstellung der

Zusammenfassung

Augenoberfläche bei Patienten mit unilateraler Stammzellinsuffizienz beitragen. Darüber hinaus könnten Haarfollikel eine leicht zugängliche Quelle adulter autologer Stammzellen mit viel versprechendem therapeutischem Potenzial für den Ersatz des Hornhautepithels und die Wiederherstellung des Sehvermögens bei Patienten mit bilateralen Erkrankungen der Augenoberfläche darstellen.

2. Introduction

2.1. Corneal epithelial cells and their niche

The cornea of the eye is composed of three layers - an outer stratified, rapidly regenerating epithelium, the underlying stroma, and an inner single-cell layered endothelium. Homeostasis of corneal epithelial cells is a basic prerequisite not only for the integrity of the ocular surface but also for corneal transparency and visual function. The continuous renewal of the corneal epithelium is provided by a population of stem cells (SC) located in the transitional zone between cornea and conjunctiva, known as the limbus, through generation of transient amplifying cells (TAC) that proliferate, migrate, and differentiate to replace lost corneal epithelial cells [1,2] (Fig.1).

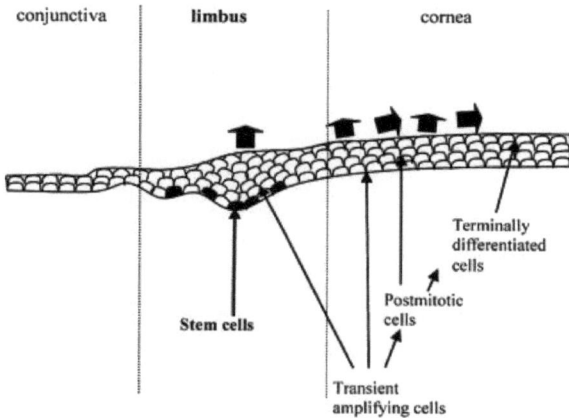

Fig.1 Location of limbal stem cells (SC) and progenitor cells. SC (black) are exclusively localized in the basal limbal epithelium. Transient amplifying cells (TAC) reside in the basal epithelia of limbus and peripheral cornea and terminally differentiated cells are arranged in the suprabasal and superficial layers of the corneal epithelium [3].

The location of corneal SC in the basal layer of the limbal epithelium is based on characteristic criteria, including slow cell cycle, the ability to retain labelled DNA precursors over a prolonged period of time, high proliferative potential and the ability for self-renewal, which also apply to other types of SC [4]. Other features that allow to distinguish limbal SC from their more differentiated progeny refer to morphologic characteristics, such as a small size averaging

10.1±0.8 µm in comparison to TAC measuring 17.1±0.8 µm [5]. Furthermore, electron microscopic analyses revealed limbal SC to possess features of immature cells like a high nuclear-cytoplasmic ratio, euchromatin-rich nuclei with barely detectable nucleoli, and a cytoplasm lacking pronounced cell organells [3].

Over the last few years some progress has been made towards finding reliable markers that may distinguish SC from their more specialized progeny TAC on the light microscopic level. Although a number of potential markers have been proposed, their role in specific identification of limbal SC is still disputable. Up to now, there seems to be no single reliable limbal SC marker. Therefore, a combined use of tissue-specific differentiation markers and putative SC or progenitor cell markers is generally applied [6]. Reports from the literature as well as our own data have shown that the basal stem and progenitor cell clusters at the limbus express the ATP binding cassette transporter ABCG2 (BCRP1), cytokeratins (K) K15 and K19, the polycomb ring finger oncogen Bmi-1, the single-pass transmembrane receptor Notch-1, and the transcription factor, p63 and its isoform p63α. In contrast, these clusters are negative for K3/K12, a marker of corneal epithelial differentiation, and proteins involved in cell-cell contacts like Connexin43 or Desmoglein-3 [3]. Consistently, the combination of differentiation-associated markers (e.g. K3/K12, Connexin43 or Desmoglein-3) and putative SC-associated markers (e.g. ABCG2, K15, p63α or Bmi-1) at present appears to be the best approach for the immunohistological identification of human limbal SC *in situ*.

The limbus is a specialized region, which is highly vascularised, innervated and also protected from potential damage by UV-light by the presence of melanin pigmentation [7]. The limbal palisades of Vogt, the site of corneal SC, form an undulating network which harbours stem and progenitor cells organized in small clusters within the basal epithelial layer, in close spatial relationship with specific basement membrane (BM) components, blood vessels as well as stromal fibroblasts. This distinct anatomical aspect may allow stem and progenitor cells to be provided with increased levels of nutrients and blood-borne growth and survival factors [3, 8-10]. SC maintenance and function are controlled by various intrinsic and extrinsic factors provided by a unique local microenvironment termed SC niche [10]. Common components of such SC niches are signalling molecules and growth factors from neighbouring cells as well as specialized extracellular matrices, which regulate cell phenotype and behaviour through cell-matrix interactions [11, 12].

The BM, forming a part of the extracellular matrix, underlies the basal epithelial cell layer of the cornea and limbus and provides structural support and anchorage for the cells. Over the past few years, it has become increasingly evident that the tissue-specific components of BM are involved in a wide spectrum of biological processes including cell growth, proliferation, differentiation and migration via cell-matrix interactions mediated by cell surface receptors [13]. Besides, BM is capable of storing and sequestering growth factors and cytokines and regulating their local concentration and release according to the respective requirements. The BM of the limbal epithelium shows specific positive immuno-labeling for type IV collagen α1 and α2 chains, laminin α5, β2, and γ1 chains, nidogen-1 and -2, as well as thrombospondin-4 as compared to that of the corneal epithelium. Differences in the BM composition of limbal and corneal epithelia suggest an influence of the BM on different cellar phenotypes and proliferative behaviour of these two cell populations. The pronounced heterogeneity of the BM in the limbal area appears to be involved in providing a unique environment for corneal stem and progenitor cells [9].

Regarding the involvement of different growth and survival factors, three patterns of cytokine interactions between epithelial and stromal cells of the cornea and limbus were described. The first group of cytokines – transforming growth factor α (TGF α), interleukin-1β, platelet-derived growth factor BB (PDGF-BB) - is released by corneal epithelial cells to act on stromal keratocytes. The second group comprising keratinocyte growth factor (KGF) and hepatocyte growth factor (HGF) is secreted by limbal and corneal fibroblasts to stimulate limbal and corneal epithelial cells, respectively [11]. The last group, including insulin like growth factor 1 (IGF-1), transforming growth factor (TGF) β1 and β2 as well as basic fibroblast growth factor (FGF-2) were found to stimulate both epithelial and fibroblast activities.

In addition, certain members of the neurotrophin family of growth factors together with their specific receptors are also present in the human limbal but not corneal epithelium. Nerve growth factor (β-NGF) is selectively expressed in the human limbal basal epithelium, together with its high-affinity receptor TrkA and its low-affinity receptor p75NTR [14]. NGF and TrkA were also found to co-localize with stem cell-associated molecular markers (ABCG-2 and p63) in the human limbal basal epithelium, but not with the corneal differentiation marker K3/K12. These observations suggest that NGF may function as an importatnt autocrine or paracrine factor supporting SC maintenance in the limbal SC niche [14, 15].

Consistently, the existing data suggest that the regulation of cellular function and gene expression of stem and differentiated cells may be influenced by the specific composition of the BM or by soluble factors secreted by the surrounding niche cells. Identification of further specific niche parameters may not only help understanding limbal SC regulation, but also improve their selective enrichment and *ex vivo* expansion in view of future therapeutic approaches.

2.2. Current therapies for unilateral/bilateral limbal stem cell deficiency

Damage to or dysfunction of the limbal SC population due to different inherited or acquired conditions, such as chemical burn or mechanical injury, results in limbal SC deficiency, which has severe consequences for ocular surface integrity and visual function. Following to a partial or total depletion of limbal epithelial SC affecting either one eye (unilateral) or both eyes (bilateral), the neighbouring conjunctival epithelium migrates over the surface of the cornea causing vascularisation, recurrent epithelial erosion, pain and ultimately blindness. Corneal blindness is a condition currently affecting about 10 million people worldwide [16, 17].

2.2.1 Unilateral stem cell deficiency

One currently used therapeutic strategy for unilateral ocular surface reconstruction is the transplantation of autologous epithelial cell sheets engineered from limbal epithelial cells expanded *ex vivo* using appropriate delivery systems, such as amniotic membrane or fibrin gel [18, 19]. This therapeutic approach usually requires a limbal biopsy from the patients´ healthy contralateral eye.

Although successful repopulation of the ocular surface with cultured limbal epithelial cells has been described for up to one year after transplantation, other studies indicate that epithelial viability is not sustained for longer periods [20] and that there is no survival of donor cells beyond 9 months after transplantation [21, 22]. This failure might arise from the depletion of SC in culture due to improper culture conditions. In most cases, the methods used to establish the cultures do not support the preservation of SC, e.g. explant cultures or air-lift cultures, which promote proliferation and terminal differentiation of TAC, but not maintenance of SC [23]. The long-term restoration of the damaged ocular surface, however, requires the preservation of limbal SC during the culture process and post-grafting [6, 24]. However, the question whether the transplanted cell sheets actually contain SC has not been clarified yet.

Since the pioneering work of Rheinwald & Green (1975) [25], studies have shown that long-term survival and serial expansion of skin epithelial SC are possible if co-cultured with fibroblast feeder cells [26]. Clonal analysis of human keratinocytes cultured on feeder layers has identified three types of clonogenic cells, giving rise to holoclones, meroclones, and paraclones [27]. Holoclone-forming cells have all the hallmarks of SC, including self-renewing capacity and a large proliferative potential, while meroclones and paraclones are generated by different stages of TAC with a limited capacity for proliferation. This discovery was followed by the identification of holoclone-forming cells in the limbal epithelium and the development of a culture system that involves enrichment of limbal SC by clonal growth on a feeder layer before seeding onto fibrin gels to produce epithelial sheets [18, 28]. Consistently, keratinocytes cultured using this method have been used to permanently restore massive skin epithelial defects caused by burns, whereas the widespread use of this very promising culture technique for the reconstruction of the ocular surface has been obviously hampered by lack of a standardized cultivation protocol [29-32].

2.2.2. Bilateral stem cell deficiency

In patients with bilateral total limbal SC deficiency, autologous limbal biopsies can not be used for the reconstruction of the ocular surface. In these cases, allogenic limbal epithelium, harvested from either living related donors or from cadaveric donor eyes, may be used for transplantation in combination with prolonged systemic immunosuppressive therapy. This approach has a very low success rate on long term, as compared with autologous cells, and immunosuppressants are not always well tolerated by patients. Therefore, present research activities focus on the evaluation of alternative autologous SC sources for *ex vivo* culture and transplantation avoiding the risk of immune-mediated rejection and the need for immunosuppression.

Regarding alternative autologous SC sources for patients suffering from bilateral limbal SC deficiency, oral mucosal epithelium has recently attracted much attention. Transplantation of cultivated oral mucosal epithelial cell sheets has provided favourable early results in patients with bilateral SC deficiency [33, 34]. Long-term clinical outcomes were, however, less satisfactory, mostly due to a relatively high rate of peripheral corneal neovascularization [35].

Another alternative autologous source of adult SC may be provided by the conjunctival epithelium. So far, cultivation and transplantation of conjunctival epithelial cell sheets have been exclusively performed in animal models of limbal SC deficiency [36, 37]. In spite of satisfying results concerning regression of corneal neovascularisation and opacity this treatment approach has not yet been adopted for the treatment of patients in the clinical setting. This may result from a potential risk of goblet cell formation, which would interfere with corneal transparency and visual function.

Therefore, further alternative SC-based therapeutic strategies for ocular surface repair and reconstruction in patients with bilateral corneal disease are still required.

2.3. Objectives: Optimization of culture conditions and search for alternative autologous stem cell sources

One emerging surgical strategy for restoring a normal corneal epithelial surface in patients with limbal SC deficiency is transplantation of *ex vivo* expanded limbal epithelial SC which represents one of the few adult human SC therapies being currently employed. In unilaterally affected patients, this therapeutic approach commonly involves the harvest of a small limbal biopsy from the patient's contralateral healthy eye followed by cell expansion *ex vivo* to generate an epithelial sheet on a transplantable carrier such as amniotic membrane or fibrin gel. Although successful restoration of the ocular surface occurs in the early postoperative period, the long-term outcome is less satisfactory, most probably due to depletion of limbal SC in culture. In patients with bilateral limbal SC deficiency, cadaveric donor eyes or alternative autologous SC sources such as oral mucosa or conjunctiva are required which, however, have provided less satisfactory long-term clinical outcomes so far. Therefore, present research activities focus on the evaluation of further alternative autologous SC sources for *ex vivo* culture and transplantation avoiding the risk of immune-mediated rejection or the need for immunosuppression.

Since the long-term clinical outcome of the currently employed limbal SC therapies has not yet been proved satisfactory, the major objective of this work was in general to establish novel SC-based cultivation techniques for therapeutic applications in patients with unilateral or bilateral limbal SC deficiency. In particular, the purpose of this study was (1) to provide an optimized culture method supporting the preferential expansion and maintenance of limbal SC throughout the cultivation process and (2) to explore the suitability of hair follicle (HF) as an alternative autologous SC source and the potential of HF to transdifferentiate into corneal epithelial-like cells when exposed to a specific microenvironment.

In order to provide an optimized culture protocol for limbal SC, the effect of several culture variables, such as limbal biopsy regions, dissociation methods, culture media as well as calcium, serum and growth factor concentrations, on clonal growth and differentiation of limbal SC was systematically analysed. Maintenance of SC phenotype within the cultivated epithelial cell sheets was evaluated by means of morphological and immunohistochemical methods using antibodies against established SC markers.

In order to investigate the capacity of HF epithelial SC to transdifferentiate into a corneal epithelial-like phenotype, HF-derived SC were exposed to cornea- or limbus-specific microenvironmental factors, such as specific extracellular matrix components or soluble growth and survival factors contained within conditioned media of tissue-specific fibroblasts. Cellular phenotype and differentiation of cultured cell sheets were evaluated by means of histological, molecular and immunohistochemical methods using antibodies against SC and tissue-specific differentiation markers.

3. Materials and Methods

3.1. Animals, tissues and cell lines

3.1.1. Animals

- C57Bl/6 mice 3-5 week old (Charles River, Sulzfeld, Germany, www.charlesriver.de)
- New Zealand white rabbits (Charles River)

3.1.2. Tissues

All human tissues used in this work were obtained after informed consent by the patients or by the relatives of the organ donors.

Corneal and limbal tissue

Human

Whole corneas for research purposes were obtained from donors if the tissue was not suitable for transplantation. Small limbal biopsies (2 mm^2) were obtained from normal donor corneas (mean age 72±14 years; 58-86 year old) subjected to corneal transplantation. Biopsies were taken from posterior, inferior, temporal und nasal limbus.

Bovine

Whole bovine (calf) corneas were obtained from a local slaughterhouse.

Hair follicles

Murine vibrissae hair follicles

Murine vibrissae hair follicles (HF) were obtained from the upper lip of 3-5 week old C57Bl/6 mouse pups (Charles River, Sulzfeld, Germany, www.criver.com).

Human scalp hair follicles

Human HF were isolated from small human scalp biopsies (0.25 cm^2) obtained during surgical intervention in the Department of Neurosurgery.

3.1.3. Cell lines

Swiss albino mouse 3T3 fibroblasts (ACC 173; DSMZ, Braunschweig, Germany, www.dsmz.de) were used as a 3T3 feeder layer for clonal expansion and growth assays of limbal and HF stem and progenitor cells.

3.2. Chemicals and expendable materials

3.2.1. Chemicals

- Acetone (Sigma-Aldrich, Munich, Germany, www.sigmaaldrich.com)
- Amphotericin B (Invitrogen, Karlsruhe, Germany, www.invitrogen.com)
- Aprotinin (Roche, Rotkreuz, Switzerland, www.roche-applied-science.com)
- Cell strainer 40µm (Schwalbach, Germany, www.millipore.com)
- DAPI (4´,6´-diamino-2-phenylindole (Sigma-Aldrich)
- Deoxycholate (DOC) (Roche)
- Eosin (Division Chroma, Münster, Germany)
- Epoxy resin (Epon 812, Fluka, Buchs Germany, www.fluka.de)
- Fibrin and Thrombin Solutions (Tissucol; Baxter-BioPharma Solutions, Halle, Germany, http://www.baxterbiopharmasolutions.com)
- Fibronectin (BD Biosciences, Heidelberg, Germany, www.bdbiosciences.com
- Gentamycin (Invitrogen)
- Glutaraldehyde (Sigma-Aldrich)
- HCl-alcohol (Carl Roth GmbH, Karlsruhe, Germany, www.roth.de)
- Hematoxilin (Division Chroma)
- Ketanest[R]S (Pfizer, Karlsruhe, Germany, www.pfizer.com)
- Laminin-1 (BD Biosciences)
- Laminin-5 (Millipore)
- Lead-citrate (Leica, Wetzler, Germany, www.leica.de)
- L-glutamin (Invitrogen)
- Magnesium chloride (Sigma-Aldrich)
- Mitomycin C (Roche)
- Natrium chloride (Sigma-Aldrich)
- Normal goat serum (Dako, Hamburg, Germany, www.dakousa.com)
- Nylon sutures, needles (Serag Wiessner, Naila, Germany, www.serag.de)
- Ofloxacin ointment (Sanofi-Aventis, Paris, France, www.sanofiaventis.com)
- Paraformaldehyde (Sigma-Aldrich)
- Penicillin (Invitrogen)
- Phosphate-buffered saline (PBS) (Sigma-Aldrich)
- Propidium iodide (Sigma-Aldrich)
- Rompun (Bayer, Leverkusen, Germany, www.bayer.de)
- Rhodamin B (Sigma-Aldrich)
- Sodium dodecyle sulfate (SDS) (Roche)
- Streptomycin (Invitrogen)
- Tergitol (Nonidet NP-40) (Roche)

- Triton X-100 (Sigma-Aldrich)
- 0.25 % trypsin-0.02% EDTA (Invitrogen)
- Type IV collagen (BD Biosciences)
- Vectashield mounting medium (Vector Laboratories, Peterborough, U.K., www.vectorlabs.com)
- Versene (Invitrogen)
- Uranyl acetate (Agar Scientific LTD, Stansted, Essex, U.K.)

3.2.2. Enzymes

- Collagenase A (Roche)
- Dispase II (Roche)
- Thermolysin (250 µg/ml) (Sigma-Aldrich)

3.2.3. Culture media and wares

Culture media
- Defined Keratinocyte Serum-Free medium with supplement (D-KSFM) (Invitrogen)
- Dulbecco´s modified Eagle´s medium (DMEM) (Invitrogen)
- Dulbecco´s modified Eagle´s medium (DMEM) without calcium (HyClone, U.S., www.hyclone.com)
- EpiLife (Invitrogen)
- Ham´s F12 (Invitrogen)
- Ham´s F12 without calcium (HyClone)
- MCDB151 (Invitrogen)
- Progenitor Cell Targeting (PCT) Cnt-20 with supplement, (CellnTec, Bern, Switzerland, www.cellntec.com)

Culture wares
- Culture flasks (BD Biosciences)
- Fetal calf serum (Invitrogen)
- Human Corneal Growth supplement (HCGS) (Invitrogen)
- Glass chamber slides (Nunc, Langenselbold, Germany, http://www.nunc.de)
- 6-well plastic dishes (Corning, N.Y, U.S.A, www.corning.com)

3.2.4. Growth factors

- Artemin (Millipore)
- Basic fibroblast growth factor (FGF) (R&D Systems, Heidelberg, Germany, www.rndsystems.com)
- Brain-derived neurotrophic factor (BDNF) (Millipore)
- Epidermal growth factor (Millipore)
- Glial cell-derived neurotrophic factor (GDNF) (Millipore)
- Insulin-like growth factor-I (IGF-I)
- Keratinocyte growth factor (KGF) (Millipore)
- Leukemia inhibitory factor (LIF) (Millipore)
- Nerve growth factor (ß-NGF) (Millipore)
- Platelet-derived growth factor-BB (PDGF-BB) (Millipore)
- Stem cell factor (SCF) (Millipore)
- Transforming growth factor-α (TGF-α) (Millipore)

3.2.5. Antibodies

For immunohistochemical, Western blot and FACS analyses performed on limbal and HF tissue and cells, the following primary and secondary antibodies summarized below were used:

Primary antibodies

Antigen	Marker	Dilution	Specificity	Company
K15	Cytokeratin 15; putative stem cell marker	1:50	human, mouse	Abcam; Cambridge, U.K.
K19	Cytokeratin 19; basal epithelial cell marker	1:50	human	Millipore; Schwalbach, Germany
Bmi-1	Polycomb ring finger oncogene; putative stem cell marker	1:500	human	Abcam; Cambridge, U.K.
P63	Transcription factor; proliferation marker	1:100	human	Abcam; Cambridge, U.K.
P63α	Stem-cell specific isoform of p63	1:100	human	Cell Signalling Technology; Danvers, MA, USA
ABCG-2	ATP-binding cassette transporter; putative stem cell marker	1:20	human	Kamiya Medical Company; Tokyo, Japan

Materials and Methods

Notch-1	Single-pass transmembrane receptor; putative stem cell marker	1:200	human	Developmental Studies Hybridoma Bank; Iowa, USA
Desmoglein-3	Transmembrane glycoprotein component of desmosomes; differentiation marker	1:25	human	Invitrogen, Zymed Laboratories; Karlsruhe, Germany
K12 (L-20)	Cytokeratin 12; corneal differentiation marker	1:50	human	Santa Cruz; Santa Cruz, CA, USA
K12 (L-15)	Cytokeratin 12; corneal differentiation marker	1:50	mouse	Santa Cruz; Santa Cruz, CA, USA
K10	Cytokeratin 10; epidermal differentiation marker	1:50	human	Santa Cruz; Santa Cruz, CA, USA
K10	Cytokeratin 10; epidermal differentiation marker	1:100	mouse	Abcam; Cambridge, U.K
K3/K12	Cytokeratins 3 and 12; corneal differentiation markers	1:1000	human	Millipore; Schwalbach, Germany
K3/K76	Cytokeratin 3/76; corneal differentiation marker	1:50	human, mouse	Millipore; Schwalbach, Germany
Pax6	Paired box gene 6 transcription factor	1:100	mouse	Abcam; Cambridge, U.K
Pax6	Paired box gene 6, transcription factor	1:150	human	Millipore; Schwalbach, Germany
α6 integrin (CD49f)	Transmembrane adhesion protein	1:50	human, mouse	Millipore; Schwalbach, Germany
β-Actin	House keeping gene	1:10.000	human	Sigma-Aldrich, Munich, Germany
β-Actin	House keeping gene	1:1000	mouse	Abcam; Cambridge, U.K

Secondary antibodies

- Alexa 488- or Alexa 555-conjugated secondary antibodies goat anti-mouse, rabbit anti-mouse and donkey anti-goat IgG (H+L) (Invitrogen-Molecular Probes, Karlsruhe, Germany, http://probes.invitrogen.com)

Materials and Methods

- Horseradish peroxidase-conjugated secondary antibodies goat anti-mouse and donkey anti-rabbit and donkey anti-goat IgG (H+L) (Pierce, Schwerte, Germany, http://www.piercenet.com)

Antibody used for FACS analysis

Rat anti-mouse α6 integrin-FITC-conjugated CD49f (BD Biosciences)

3.2.6. Primers

For mRNA analyses performed on murine and human HF tissue by means of real time RT-PCR, the following primers were used:

Gene product	Sequence (5´-3´)	Accession number
mK10	AGTGGTACGAGAAGCATGGCAAC CATTGTCAGTTGTCAGGGTGAGG	NM_010660
mK12	GCAGGAGATAGTGAATGGCGAAGTG TGCTAACAAGACCCAACCTGCATAG	NM_010661
mPax6	AGGGCCAAATGGAGAAGAGAAG CCAACATGGAACCTGATGTGAA	NM_013627
mß-actin	GTGACGTTGACATCCGTAAAGACC GGAGCCAGAGCAGTAATCTCCTTC	NM_007393
hK10	CCTGGCATTGTCGATCTGAA GCTGGAAGGCAAAATCAAGG	NM_000421
hK12	GATGAGACCACCTCACCATTCAC GTGACAGACTCCAAATCACAAGCAC	NM_000223
hK15	CTCTCTTGTGGGAAGAAACCAC GGCTCAGAACCAGGAGTACAAG	NM_002275
hPax6	GGTATCATAACTCCGCCCATTC ACAGCCCTCACAAACACCTACA	NM_000280
hß-actin	AGTGGGGTGGCTTTTAGGAT ACTGGAACGGTGAAGGTGAC	NM_001101

m: murine; h: human

MWG Biotech (Ebersberg, Germany, http://www.eurofinsdna.com)

3.2.7. Kits

- Micro BCA Protein Assay kit (Perbio Science, Bonn Germany, http://www.perbio.com)
- RNeasy kit (Quiagen, Hilden, Germany, http://www1.qiagen.com)
- SYBR Green Supermix (Biorad)

3.2.8. Surgical instruments

- Forceps and Scissors (extra fine) (Geuder AG, Heidelberg, Germany)
- Graefe nifes (F.S.T., Heidelberg, Germany)
- Suture tweezers (Geuder AG, Heidelberg, Germany, www.geuder.de)
- Trephines (difa Cooper S.P.A., Caronno, Italy)
- Vannas scissors (F.S.T., Heidelberg, Germany)

3.3. Equipment and software

3.3.1. Equipment

- (ChemiLucent) (Chemicon, Germany)
- Chemi-Smart 5000 chmiluminescence detection system and software (Vilber Lourmat, Eberhardtzell, Germany)
- Electron microscope EM 906E (Leo, Oberkochen, Germany)
- Digital camera ColorView I (Olympus Optical Co., Hamburg, Germany, www.olympus.de)
- Fluorescence microscope BX51 (Olympus)
- MoFlo cell sorter (Cytomation, Frieburg, Germany, http://www.cytomation-bioinstrument.com
- 12-bit monochrome CCD camera F-View II (Olympus)
- Power supply Power Pac Basic (Biorad, Munich, Germany, www.biorad.de)
- Prism 3100 DNA sequencer; Applied Biosystems, Inc. [ABI], Germany, http://www3.appliedbiosystems.com)
- Semidry transfer cell Transblot SD (Biorad)
- Spectral photometer SLT Spectra (SLT Labinstruments Germany, www.labinstruments.de)
- Stereomicroscope (Novex, Amsterdam, Netherlands, www.novex.com)
- Thermal cycler and software (MyIQ; Bio-Rad, München, Germany, http://www.bio-rad.com)
- Thermostat Plus (Eppendorf, Hamburg, Germany, www.eppendorf.com)
- Vertical electrophoresis cell MiniProtean 3 (Biorad)

3.3.2. Software

- Cell^F (Olympus Soft Imaging Solutions GmbH, Münster, Germany, www.olympus.de)
- Primer 3 software for primer design available at:
  (http://www-genome.wi.mit.edu/genome_software/other/primer3.html)
- SPSS 15.0 (SPSS Inc. Chicago, Illinois, USA)

3.4. Cell culture

3.4.1. Dissociation and separation methods

Limbal epithelial cells

Small biopsies were taken from superior limbus using a scalpel and fine scissors and four different methods of SC isolation from limbal tissue specimens were compared:

1. Specimens were incubated in dispase II solution (2.4 U/ml) for 1.5 hours at 37°C followed by incubation in 0.25 % trypsin-0.02% EDTA for 10 min. at 37°C to obtain single cell suspensions.
2. Specimens were minced and directly incubated in 0.25% trypsin-0.02% EDTA for 1.5 hours at 37°C under continuous agitation by 700 rpm on Thermostat Plus
3. Specimens were minced and directly incubated in 0.25 % trypsin-0.02% EDTA for 1.5 hours at room temperature under continuous magnetic stirring at a speed of 500-700 rpm.
4. Specimens were treated with thermolysin (250 µg/ml) for 1.5 hours at 37°C followed by incubation in 0.25 % trypsin-0.02% EDTA for 10 min. at 37°C to obtain single cell suspensions.

Hair follicle cells

To isolate murine HF, the upper lip containing the pads with the vibrissae was dissected and its inner surface was exposed. The subcutaneous fat and the connective tissue were carefully removed and the vibrissae were then pulled away from the pad using a fine forceps under a dissecting microscope. The HF together with its surrounding collagen capsule was cut into three fragments (Fig. 10A,B). The first transversal cut was made just below the sebaceous gland. The second cut was made at the site of insertion of the nerve fibres, which is proximal to the site of inferior enlargement of the outer root sheath. Each fragment was then separately transferred into a 35 mm dish containing 1 ml of collagenase A/dispase II (1 mg/ml) and incubated for 30 min at 37°C. After complete digestion of the collagen capsule, the HF fragments were transferred into fresh cell culture dishes containing 0.05% trypsin and incubated for about 1.5 hours until cell dissociation was completed.

To isolate human HF, they were dissected from the surrounding dermis and fat tissue under a dissecting microscope. The dissection of the stem cell-containing bulge region and the dissociation of the bulge cells was performed as described above for murine HF.

3.4.1.1. Fluorescence-activated cell sorting

Freshly isolated murine HF cells were suspended in PBS-EDTA (5mM) and stained with α6 integrin-FITC-conjugated CD49f antibody diluted 1:100 for 30 min on ice. Following three washing steps in PBS-EDTA, α6 integrin–positive and –negative cells were isolated using a MoFlo cell sorter and expanded on a 3T3 feeder cell layer.

3.4.2. Cell culture under various culture conditions

3T3 fibroblasts
Swiss albino mouse 3T3 fibroblasts were grown in Dulbecco´s Modified Eagle medium (DMEM) with 4500g/l glucose and supplemented with 10% FCS, 10.000 U/ml penicillin, 10.000 µg/ml streptomycin, and 25 µg/ml amphotericin B. When the cells reached approximately 80% confluence they were passaged at a ratio 1:25 and seeded into fresh 250 ml culture flasks. The passaging followed every three days and the cells were incubated at 37°C under 5% CO_2 and 95% humidity.

Limbal epithelial cells
As a standard protocol single cell suspensions were obtained from biopsies taken from superior limbus using a combined dispase II/trypsin-EDTA (ethylenediaminetetraaceticacid) treatment (see above, chapter 3.4.1. procedure 1). The cell suspensions were seeded at a density of 1 x 10^3 cells/cm^2 on a 3T3 feeder cell layer in 6-well culture plates. Cell cultures were incubated at 37°C under 5% CO_2 and 95% humidity in different culture media (see below) with medium MCDB151 containing Human Corneal Growth Supplement (HCGS), 5ng/ml human Epidermal Growth Factor (EGF), 10% fetal calf serum (FCS), and 5 µg/ml gentamycin (medium 1) used as the standard medium. The medium was changed every 2-3 days.

For culture of limbal epithelial cells, five different culture media were compared:
1. MCDB151 containing 0.03 mmol/L calcium and supplemented with HCGS containing 0.18 µg/ml hydrocortisone, 5 µg/ml insulin, 5 µg/ml transferrin, 1 ng/ml EGF, and 0.2% bovine pituitary extract.
2. Equal parts of Dulbecco´s modified Eagle´s medium and Ham´s F12 medium (DMEM/F12) containing 1.2 mmol/L calcium and supplemented with HCGS.
3. Defined Keratinocyte Serum-Free medium (D-KSFM) containing < 0.1 mmol/L calcium and D-KSFM supplement of unknown composition.
4. Progenitor Cell Targeting medium (PCT) CnT-20 containing 0.07 mmol/L calcium and Cnt-20 supplement of unknown composition.
5. EpiLife medium containing 0.06 mmol/L calcium and supplemented with HCGS.

All media were supplemented with different concentrations (0-20%) of FCS as well as different concentrations (0-20 ng/ml) of EGF to test their effect on the clonal growth of limbal stem and progenitor cells.

To further evaluate the effect of growth factors other than EGF, serum-free MCDB151 medium was supplemented with one of the following growth factors, all at a concentration of 10 ng/ml: transforming growth factor-α (TGF-α), keratinocyte growth factor (KGF), platelet-derived growth factor-BB (PDGF-BB), leukemia inhibitory factor (LIF), hepatocyte growth factor (HGF), stem cell factor (SCF), insulin-like growth factor-I (IGF-I), and basic fibroblast growth factor (FGF). Neurotrophic factors, including brain-derived neurotrophic factor (BDNF), nerve growth factor (ß-NGF), glial cell-derived neurotrophic factor (GDNF), and artemin, all at concentrations of 100 ng/ml, were also included in the analysis.

Murine and human hair follicle cells

Basic culture medium for murine and human HF epithelial cells was prepared containing three parts of DMEM and one part of Ham's F12 medium (0.4 mM Ca^{2+}) (HyClone) supplemented with 10% FCS, 10 ng/ml EGF, 500 mg/l L-glutamin, and HCGS (0.2% bovine pituitary extract, 0.18 µg/ml hydrocortisone, 5 µg/ml insulin and 5 µg/ml transferrin) as well as 10.000 U/ml penicillin, 10.000 µg/ml streptomycin, 25 µg/ml amphotericin B. Cell suspensions were seeded either on a 3T3 feeder cell layer or on fibrin gels and incubated for two weeks at 37°C under 5% CO_2 and 95% humidity.

3.4.3. Clonal expansion on a 3T3 feeder cell layer

The clonal expansion of stem and progenitor cells was performed on a 3T3 feeder cell layer. When 80% confluence was reached, 3T3 cells were growth arrested with 4 µg/ml mitomycin C for two hours at 37°C, washed, harvested with 0.25% trypsin-0.02% EDTA and plated onto 6-well plastic dishes at a density of $2x10^4$ cells/cm^2.

Single cell suspensions of enzymatically isolated human limbal epithelial cells and human HF bulge epithelial cells were plated at a density of $1x10^3$ cells/cm^2 onto the 3T3 feeder cell layer and cultivated for 2 weeks. Clonal growth was daily monitored by contrast microscopy and analyzed on day 14 following removal of the feeder layer with 0.02% EDTA for 30 seconds, fixation in 4% paraformaldehyde and staining with 2% rhodamine B.

Clonal expansion of murine HF SC was performed on a feeder layer using three different approaches: (i) bulge explant outgrowth, (ii) single cell suspensions obtained by mechanical dissection and enzymatic digestion, and (iii) single cell suspensions obtained by fluorescence activated cell sorting (FACS).

3.5. Clonal growth assay

Colony formation on a 3T3 feeder layer was analyzed on day 14 following removal of the 3T3 cells with 0.02% EDTA for 30 seconds, fixation in 4% paraformaldehyde and staining with 2% rhodamine B. Colonies were classified into holo-, mero-, and paraclones according to their size, morphology, cell number, and cellular phenotype as originally reported [27]. Cell numbers of individual holoclones were determined using cloning cylinders (Sigma-Aldrich) and a cell counting system (CASY, Roche Innovatis, Basel, Switzerland). Colony size, defined as diameter of individual holoclones in millimeter, and colony density, defined as percentage area of the culture dish covered by all holoclones, were determined after scanning of the culture plates using an image analysis software Cell^F. The colony-forming efficiency (CFE) was calculated as the number of holo-, mero- and paraclones divided by the total number of cells seeded per well. For serial propagation, clonal cells were passaged after 14 days of culture, seeded at a density of 1×10^3 cells/cm^2 on a 3T3 feeder layer, and cultured for another 14 days.

3.6. Coating of chamber slides with extracellular matrix components

Glass chamber slides were coated with various matrix components including type IV collagen (40 μg/ml), fibronectin (20 μg/ml), laminin-1(100 μg/ml) and laminin-5 (10 μg/ml) by incubation for 1hour at room temperature. Afterwards, the slides were briefly washed with phosphate-buffered saline (PBS) and dried under a laminar flow bench before seeding of clonal cells. To prepare the appropriate concentrations of the coating substrates, the commercially acquired stock solutions were diluted using unconditioned serum-free culture medium.

3.7. Conditioning of culture medium with corneal and limbal epithelial cells and stromal fibroblasts

Conditioned media (CM) were derived from both epithelial cells and fibroblasts from human and calf corneas. Corneal buttons were dissected into central, peripheral, and limbal regions. Incubation of tissue specimens in 2.4 U/ml dispase II for 1.5 hours at 37°C was followed by mechanical separation of the corneal epithelium from the underlying stroma. The detached epithelial sheets were trypsinized in 0.25% trypsin-EDTA for 15 minutes at 37°C to obtain a single cell suspension. The remaining connective tissue was cut into small pieces and placed in 2 mg/ml collagenase A overnight at 37°C. After digestion, the epithelial cells and fibroblasts were separately seeded into cell culture flasks, and cultivated for 24 hours in DMEM:Ham´s F12 (3:1) medium (1.2 mM Ca2+) (HyClone). After cell adhesion, spreading and reaching approximately 60-80% confluence, the medium was changed to DMEM:Ham's F12 (3:1) (0.4 mM Ca2+) for another 48 hours, collected, filtered through a 40 μm cell strainer, and stored at -80°C until use. The harvested media were designated conditioned media (CM). Only the first passage (P1) of the epithelial cells and the first 3 passages (P1, P2, and P3) of freshly isolated and cultivated stromal fibroblasts were used for production of CM. In addition, CM from murine 3T3 fibroblasts was prepared as described above and used as control.

3.8. Subculture of clonal cells under various environmental conditions

Murine and human hair follicle cells
After clonal expansion on a 3T3 feeder cell layer for 14 days, the feeder layer was removed using Versene and clonal cells were trypsinized (0.25%Trypsin-EDTA) for 15 min at 37°C. Murine HF cells were seeded at a density of 1×10^5 cells/cm^2 onto glass chamber slides coated with different matrix components, or into uncoated 6 well culture plates. Murine HF cells were subcultivated for 8-16 days in human fibroblast CM obtained from either central or peripheral cornea or limbus, or from 3T3 murine fibroblasts. 3T3 cell-derived CM served as control, because primary cultures of murine keratinocytes require fibroblast CM for long-term culture [38].

Human HF cells were subcultivated for the same period of time in CM derived from either limbal, or central, or peripheral corneal fibroblasts combined with epithelial cell-derived CM from the respective region. This combination of fibroblastic and epithelial CM resulted in a considerably improved epithelial morphology of the cultured cells. Unconditioned culture medium served as negative control. Culture conditions were switched from medium-calcium concentration (0.4 mM Ca2+) to high-calcium concentration (1.2 mM Ca2+) after 7 days in order to promote differentiation. For all experiments, CM were added to the normal culture media at a ratio of 1:1.

3.9. Generation of epithelial sheets on fibrin

Fibrin gels were prepared by dissolving fibrinogen and thrombin stock solutions in 1.1% NaCl and 1 mmol/L CaCl$_2$ to a final concentration of 10 mg/ml fibrinogen and 3 IU/ml thrombin. Limbal and HF holoclones were harvested by trypsination (0.25%Trypsin-EDTA for 15 min. at 37°C), seeded on top of fibrin gels at a density of 1×10^5 cells/cm^2, and subcultivated in appriopriate conditioned or unconditioned media for 14-16 days. Limbal clonal cells were cultivated in MCDB151 medium supplementd as described above (see chapter 3.4.2.) and additionally containing 100 ng/ml β-

NGF. Murine and human HF cells were subcultured in various human or bovine CM, respectively. For limbal epithelial cells culture conditions were switched from low-calcium conditions (0.03 mmol/L Ca2+) to medium-calcium conditions (0.4 mmol/L Ca2+) after 7 days in order to promote formation of adhesion molecules. For HF cells culture conditions were switched from medium-calcium concentration (0.4 mM Ca2+) to high-calcium concentration (1.2 mM Ca2+) after 7 days for the same purpose.

3.10. Methods of evaluation

3.10.1. Light and electron microscopy

For light microscopy cultivated cells or cell sheets were fixed in 4% paraformaldehyde in 0.1M phosphate buffer, dehydrated, and embedded in paraffin. To deparaffinise the sections were treated with xylene for 10 min. in four consecutiv steps. To rehydrate the sections were immersed in graded ethanol concentrations (100%, 95%, 80%, 70%) for 5 min. in four consecutiv steps and then rinsed with distilled water. Nuclei were stained with hematoxylin for 10 min. and rinsed with water to remove excess hematoxylin. Afterwards the sections were corroded in 1% HCl-ethanol for 5 sec., then rinsed in water, treated with NH_4OH for 30 sec, and finally rinsed in distilled water. Afterwards the cytoplasm of the cells was stained with eosin by consecutively dipping the sections in the following solutions: eosin for 3´min., 5 times in HCl-ethanol for 5 min., several times in 100% ethanol for 5 min., xylene and finally acetone. Stained sections were mounted in resin.

For electron microscopic analyses cultivated cells and cell sheets were fixed in 2.5% glutaraldehyde in 0.1M phosphate buffer, postfixed in 2% buffered osmium tetroxide, dehydrated in a graded alcohol ethanol series, and embedded in epoxy resin, according to the standard protocol as previously described [3]. Ultra-thin sections of 0.1µm thickness were stained with uranyl acetate- and lead citrate for further electron microscopic examination.

3.10.2. Immunohisto-/cytochemistry

For immunohistochemical experiments tissue samples (mouse and human eyes and hair follicles) and fibrin-based cell sheets were embedded in optimal cutting temperature (OCT) compound and frozen in isopentane-cooled liquid nitrogen.
Immunocytochemistry, was performed on epithelial clones or cell sheets without fibrin carrier.
Both the cells cultured in chamber slides and 5-7 µm thick cryosections were fixed with cold acetone for 10 min. at 4°C, washed with PBS, and permeabilized with 0.1% Triton X-100 in PBS for 10 min. at 4°C. After blocking with 10% normal goat serum cells were incubated in primary

Materials and Methods

antibodies diluted in PBS for 2 h at room temperature or over night at 4°C, respectively. Antibody binding was detected by Alexa 488- or Alexa 555-conjugated secondary antibodies and nuclear counterstaining was performed with propidium iodide or DAPI (4´,6´-diamino-2-phenylindole). Slides were washed and coverslipped with Vectashield mounting medium prior to evaluation with a fluorescence microscope. In negative control experiments, the primary antibody was replaced by PBS or equimolar concentrations of an irrelevant primary antibody.

3.10.3. Real-Time RT-PCR

Total RNA was isolated using the RNeasy kit from both murine and human cells expanded under various environmental conditions. First-strand cDNA synthesis from 500 ng of total RNA and quantitative real-time PCR were performed with a thermal cycler and software MyIQ according to the standard protocol as previously described [39]. PCR reactions were run in duplicate and contained 2 µl of the 1:5 diluted first-strand cDNA, 0.4 µl each of upstream- and downstream primer, 3.0 to 4.0 mM MgCl2, and master mix (SYBR Green Supermix). The following program was used: 95°C for 3 min, and 40 cycles of 95°C for 30 s, 62°C for 30 s, and 72°C for 30 s. Human and murine exon-spanning primers were designed by means of Primer 3 software and are summarized in a table above (see above, 3.2.6.). For quantification, serially diluted standard curves of plasmid-cloned cDNA as previously described [39] were run in parallel, and amplification specificity was checked by using melting curve and sequence analyses (Prism 3100 DNA sequencer). For normalization of gene expression levels, mRNA ratios relative to the housekeeping gene β-actin were calculated.

3.10.4. Western Blot Analysis

Protein concentrations were determined using the Micro BCA Protein Assay kit with bovine serum albumin as a standard. Total protein was isolated from human and murine cells expanded under various environmental conditions using RIPA buffer (150 mM NaCl, 1% NP-40, 0.5% DOC, 0.1% SDS, 50 mM Tris pH 8, 10 µg/ml Aprotinin). 10 µg of total protein were separated by SDS-PAGE under reducing conditions, and immunoblot analyses were performed as previously described [39] using following antibodies: polyclonal goat anti-mouse K12 (L-15) (1:100, Santa Cruz), polyclonal rabbit anti-mouse K10 (Abcam, 1:100), polyclonal rabbit anti-mouse Pax6 (1:1000, Abcam), polyclonal rabbit anti-mouse β-actin (1:1000, Abcam), polyclonal goat anti-human K12 (L-20) (1:100, Santa Cruz), polyclonal goat anti-human K10 (1:100, Santa Cruz), monoclonal mouse anti-human β-actin (1:10.000, Sigma-Aldrich). Equal loading was verified with anti- β-actin antibodies. In negative control experiments, the primary antibody was replaced by PBS. Immunodetection was performed with horseradish peroxidase-conjugated secondary antibodies (Pierce) diluted 1:1000 and chemiluminescence (ChemiLucent). Signals were analysed and quantified (Chemi-Smart 5000 chmiluminescence detection system and software). For standardization of protein expression, expression levels and signal intensity ratios relative to the housekeeping gene β-actin were calculated.

3.11. Engraftment of cultivated hair follicle epithelial sheets

Generation of limbal stem cell deficiency in an animal model
Total limbal stem cell deficiency (LSCD) was created in two New Zealand white rabbit (Charles River) eyes by surgically removing the entire corneal epithelium by superficial keratectomy.

Engraftment
The fibrin-based human HF epithelial sheets cultured for two weeks in limbal fibroblast- derived CM were transplanted onto the denuded corneal surface of one eye to completely cover the resected area and sutured with 10-0 nylon sutures. A normal, untreated rabbit eye served as control. The HF graft was covered with amniotic membrane and therapeutic soft contact lenses for protection. A total tarsorrhaphy was performed with 6-0 nylon sutures.

Postoperatively, the rabbits were treated daily with topical antibiotics of 0.3% ofloxacin ointment (Sanofi-Aventis, Paris, France), and systemic antibiotics (10 mg Gentamycin/rabbit, delivered intramusculary) to inhibit a possible xenogenic reaction or non-specific inflammation.

The ocular surfaces of the rabbits were slit lamp examined by slit lamp microscopy on the day of transplantation as well as 7 days postoperatively to monitor the extent of epithelialization.

3.12. Statistics

Data are presented as the mean ± SD. Statistical evaluation of significant differences between different assays or samples was performed with the Mann-Whitney-Test for non-parametric analysis. $P < 0.05$ was considered statistically significant.

4. Results

4.1. Optimization of culture conditions for expansion of limbal stem and progenitor cells

4.1.1. Clonal growth and phenotypic characterization

When supported by growth-arrested 3T3 feeder cells, human limbal epithelial cells gave rise to macroscopic colonies within 10 to 12 days after inoculation. After 3 to 4 weeks, colonies eventually fused and generated a stratified layer. In general, the distinction among the three clonal types was based on colony morphology and size: large, nearly circular colonies (4-10mm in diamter) with smooth outline were identified as holoclones, medium sized colonies (1-4mm in diameter) with wrinkled outline as meroclones, and small, highly irregular colonies (<1mm in diameter) as paraclones (Fig. 2) [27, 40-42]. Average CFE was found to range from 0.3-0.4%. Holoclones contained 2-5 x 10^4 cells/mm^2 and consisted mainly of small cuboid, densely packed cells in a regular mosaic-like pattern, concentrated in the periphery of the colony (Fig. 2A); the center of the colony appeared stratified with the upper differentiating layers consisting of large flattened cells covering the basal layer of small cuboid cells. In contrast, most cells in meroclones and all cells in paraclones had an increased cell size and appeared flattened (Fig. 2B,C).

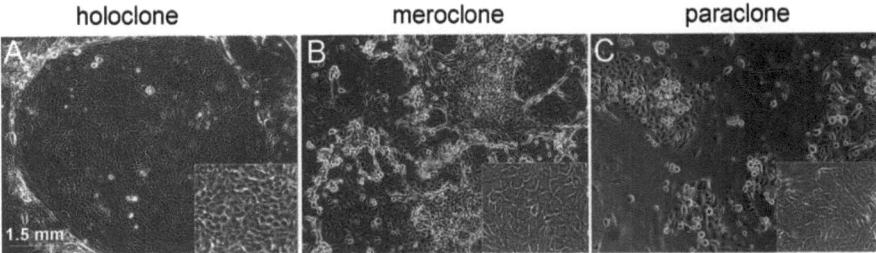

Figure 2. Clonal growth on a 3T3 feeder cell layer. The distinction between the three clonal types is based upon colony morphology and size: **(A)** holoclones: large, nearly circular colonies with smooth outline arising from stem cells. **(B)** meroclones: medium sized colonies with wrinkled outline arising from transient amplifying cells. **(C)** paraclones: small, highly irregular colonies arising from nearly terminally differentiated keratinocytes.

Results

Immunocytochemical analysis of holoclones using antibodies against known limbal stem and progenitor (p63, p63α, Bmi-1, ABCG2, K15, K19, Notch1) as well as differentiation markers (K3/K12, desmoglein-3) revealed rather differentiated cells (positive for desmoglein-3) in the suprabasal cells in the center and rather undifferentiated proliferating cells (positive for p63) in the periphery of holoclones representing a rim of intense proliferation close to the perimeter of the colony (Fig. 3A). Whereas positive nuclear p63 immunostaining was found in the majority of cells (Fig. 3B), p63α, which has been reported to be the most specific isoform and marker for holoclone identification [30, 42, 43], was restricted to peripheral small cells (Fig. 3C). There was almost no overlap between desmoglein-3 positive and p63α positive cells. Co-expression of Bmi-1 in peripheral cells (Fig. 3D) also identifies human limbal holoclones [24]. Expression of ABCG2 was observed in clusters of cells close to the clone border (Fig. 3E). Each holoclone contained one to few cells in the periphery, which showed cytoplasmic labelling for K15 (Fig. 3F) and Notch-1 (Fig. 3G). These cells were characterized by a small diameter of <10μm and a large nuclear-cytoplasmic ratio, thus potentially representing stem or progenitor cells. Cells positive for K19 were distributed throughout the basal layer of the colonies (Fig. 3H). K3/K12 immunostaining, indicative of the extent of corneal epithelial differentiation, was confined to few superficial cells in the central stratified region (Fig. 3I).

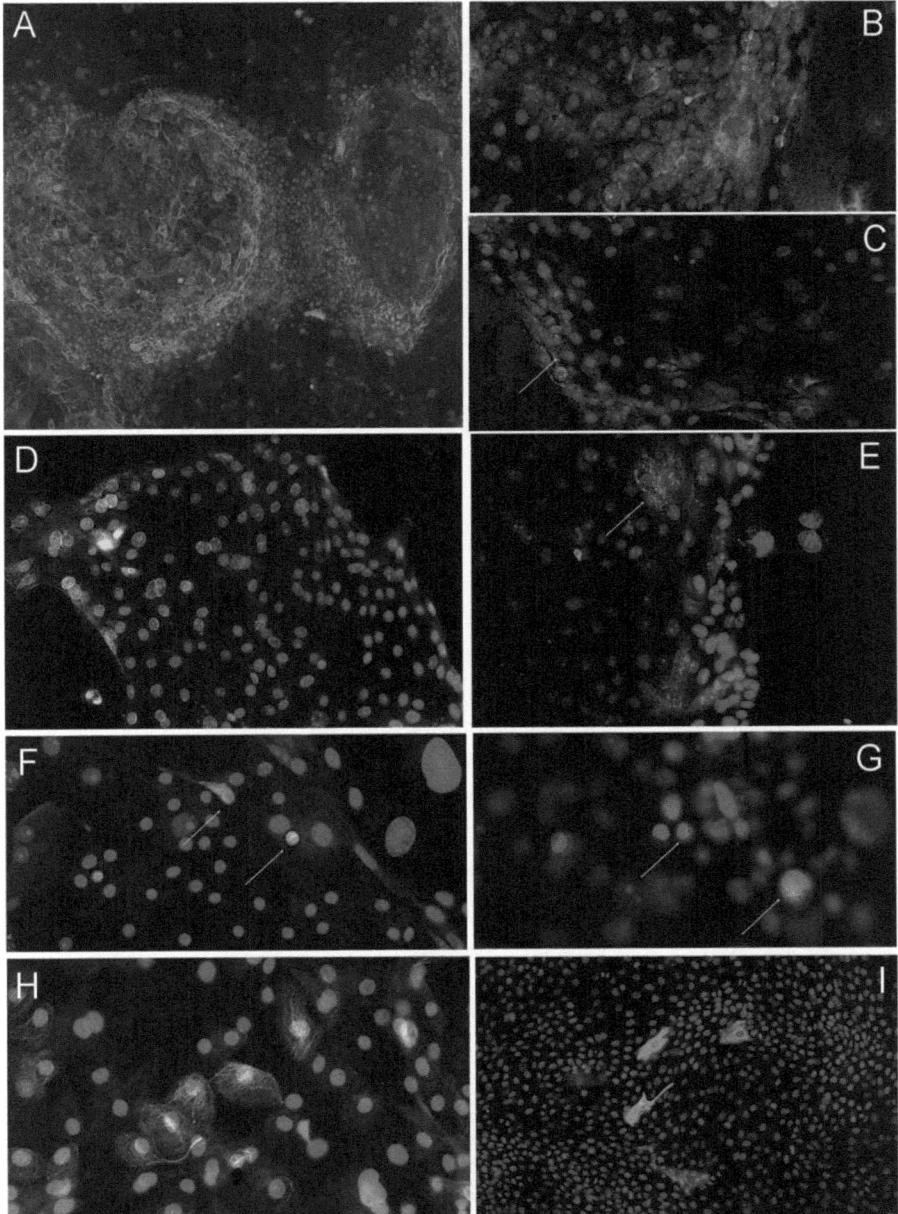

Figure 3. Phenotypic analysis of holoclones. (A-I) Immunofluorescence analysis of holoclones using antibodies against stem cell (p63, p63α, Bmi-1, ABCG2, K15, K19, Notch1) and differentiation (K3/K12, desmoglein-3) markers. (A) Double staining for desmoglein-3 (green fluorescence) and p63 (red

fluorescence) shows rather differentiated cells in the suprabasal layers in the center and rather undifferentiated proliferating cells in the periphery of holoclones. **(B)** Positive nuclear p63 immunostaining (red fluorescence) was found in the majority of cells and partly overlapped with desmoglein-3 immunostaining (green fluorescence). **(C)** The isoform p63α (red) was restricted to peripheral small, densely packed cells (arrow) negative for desmoglein-3 (green). **(D)** Expression of Bmi-1 (green) was observed in peripheral cells. **(E)** Immunopositivity for ABCG2 (green) was present in cell clusters close to the clone border (arrows). **(F)** Expression of K15 (green) was present in few cells in the periphery of the clone (arrow). **(G)** Positive staining for Notch-1 (green) was also found in few cells close to the clone border (arrows). **(H)** Cells positive for K19 (green) were distributed throughout the basal layer of the colonies. **(I)** K3/K12 immunostaining (green) was confined to few superficial cells in the central stratified region of the clone. Nuclear staining was performed with DAPI (4´,6-diamidino-2-phenylindole) (blue, **A-C**) or propidium iodide (red, **D-I**). Magnification: 100x (G,H), 40x (B-F), 20x (**A,I**)

4.1.2. Effect of limbal region and donor age on clonal growth

To evaluate the clonogenic ability of the different areas of the limbus, cells from the superior, inferior, nasal, and temporal limbus of six donor eyes (69 ± 17.1 years) were analyzed. The CFE was comparable in superior and inferior as well as in nasal and temporal regions and was markedly higher in the superior (0.4%) and inferior (0.3%) than in the nasal (0.1%) and temporal (0.1%) areas of the limbus. Consistently, colony density and colony size were significantly ($p<0.05$) larger in superior and inferior regions compared to nasal and temporal regions (Fig.4.1 A-F). Based on these observations, the superior limbus was selected as the region of tissue sampling for all further experiments.

The averaged CFE declined with the age of the donor. In patients aged 50-65 years, the CFE was 0.5-0.6%, but the CFE dropped significantly to 0.3% in patients aged 65-85 years. Colony density and size decreased from 80% and 8 mm diameter to 40% and 4mm diameter in the older age group (data not shown).

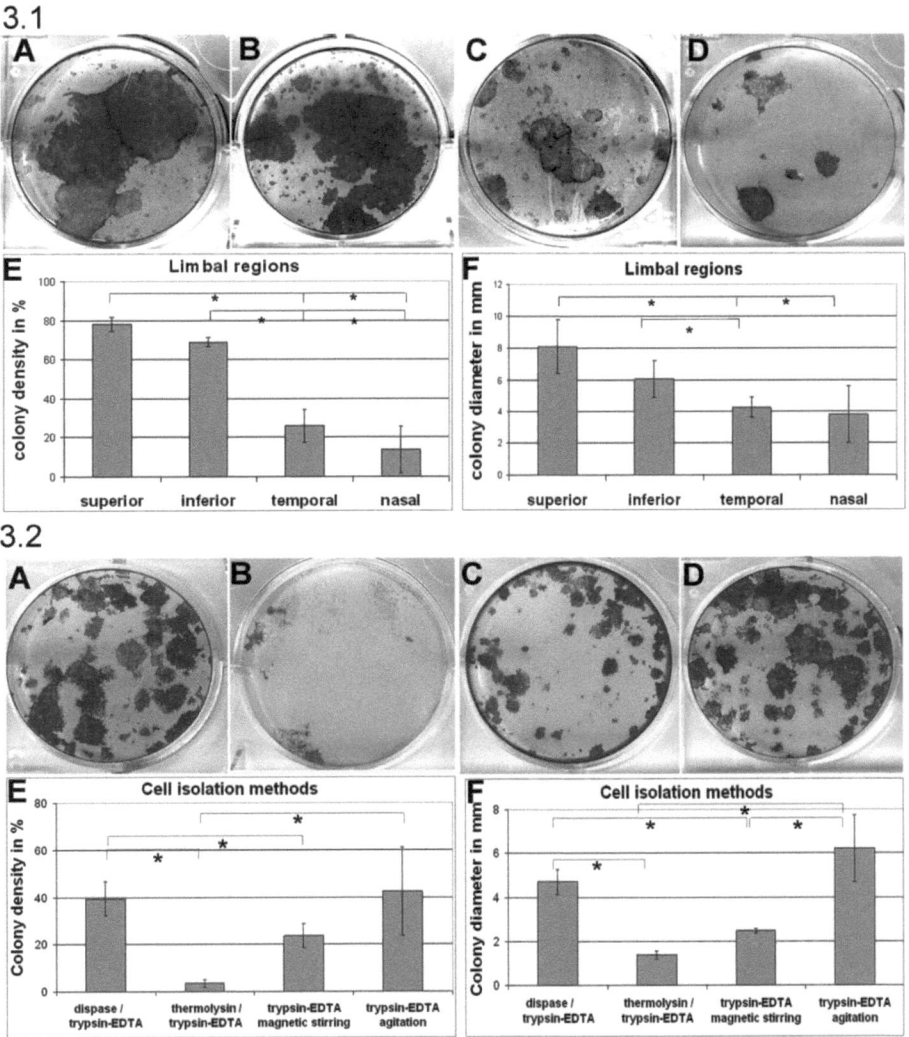

Figure 4. Effect of limbal regions and dissociation methods on clonal growth. 4.1. (A-F) Analysis of the clonogenic potential of epithelial cells isolated from different areas of the limbus (superior, inferior, temporal, nasal) and expanded on a 3T3 feeder layer for 14 days. **(A-D)** Colonies obtained from the superior **(A)**, the inferior **(B)**, the temporal **(C)**, and the nasal **(D)** regions of the limbus were stained with rhodamin B and analyzed using an image analysis software. **(E,F)** Quantitative analysis of colony density **(E)** and colony diameter **(F)** showing significantly increased clonal growth in superior and inferior regions compared to nasal and temporal regions. Values represent means ± SD of six separate experiments (*$p < 0.05$; Mann-Whitney-Test).

Results

4.2 (A-F) Analysis of the clonogenic potential of epithelial cells isolated from the superior limbus by four different enzymatic dissociation methods and expanded on a 3T3 feeder layer for 14 days. **(A-D)** Colonies obtained by combined dispase II/trypsin-EDTA digestion **(A)**, combined thermolysin/trypsin-EDTA digestion **(B)**, trypsin-EDTA and magnetic stirring **(C)**, and trypsin-EDTA with agitation **(D)** were stained with rhodamin B and analyzed using an image analysis software. **(E,F)** Quantitative analysis of colony density **(E)** and colony diameter **(F)** showing significantly increased clonal growth after dissociation with dispase II/trypsin-EDTA or trypsin-EDTA and agitation. Values represent means ± SD of four separate experiments (*p < 0.05; Mann-Whitney-Test).

4.1.3. Effect of dissociation method on clonal growth

To establish the most effective method of SC isolation from small biopsies (2 mm^2) taken from the superior limbus of four pairs of donor eyes (59 ± 15.7 years), four different enzymatic dissociation methods were compared. Although the total cell yield was comparable between all methods used, amounting to approximately 1.0 x10^4 cells/mm^2 tissue, the CFE showed significant differences between dispaseII/trypsin-EDTA (0.37%), thermolysin/trypsin-EDTA (0.01%), trypsin-EDTA with magnetic stirring (0.35%), and trypsin-EDTA with agitation (0.34%). Colony density and size were highest with a combined extraction method using dispaseII/trypsin-EDTA and a single extraction method using trypsin-EDTA with agitation (p<0.05), although the coefficient of variation was greater using the latter method due to highly variable proportions of live and dead cells in the single cell suspensions (Fig. 4.2 A-F). Therefore, the combined dispaseII/trypsin-EDTA digestion method, which consistently yielded high numbers of viable cells (85-90%), was selected as the standard isolation procedure for all further experiments.

4.1.4. Effect of culture conditions on clonal growth

To evaluate the effect of culture conditions on clonal growth, we first compared five different culture media containing low (MCDB151, PCT, D-KSFM, EpiLife) or high (DMEM/F12) calcium concentrations, commonly used for *in vitro* expansion of corneal and epithelial progenitor cells. Although the CFE was comparable in all media (0.3% in MCDB151, 0.35% in PCT, 0.31 in D-KSFM, 0.4 in DMEM/F12) except EpiLife, colony growth was fastest in DMEM/F12 and slowest in MCDB151, while EpiLife did not support clonal growth at all. Consistently, cells cultured in DMEM/F12 showed a significantly higher colony density and size than that grown in MCDB151 after 2 weeks of culture (p<0.05) (Fig. 5). However, these fast-growing colonies mostly consisted of large, flattened, differentiated appearing cells, which reached senescence after 3 to 4 passages. Similarly, the colonies grown in PCT and D-KSFM revealed a rather irregular outline and pleomorphic cellular phenotype (Fig. 5). Despite of delayed growth in MCDB151, this medium produced the most regular and compact holoclones consisting of small tightly packed cells, which could be serially cultured for at least 8 passages. A prolonged culture time of 3 to 4 weeks promoted further clonal growth in MCDB151 up to complete overgrowth of the culture plate. Therefore, MCDB151 was selected as the most effective culture medium to support the growth of limbal holoclones and used as the standard medium for all further experiments.

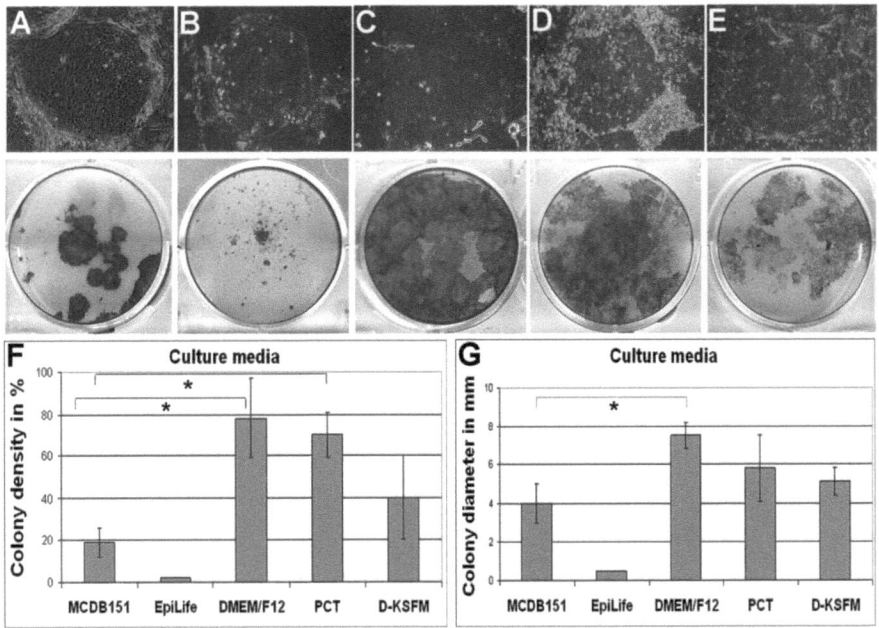

Figure 5. Effect of different cell culture media on clonal growth. (A-E) Analysis of the clonogenic potential of epithelial cells isolated from the superior limbus by dispase II/trypsin-EDTA and expanded on a 3T3 feeder layer for 14 days in MCDB151 (A), EpiLife (B), DMEM/F12 (C), PCT (D), and D-KSFM (E) supplemented with HCGS, 10% FCS and 5 ng/ml EGF. Analysis of clone morphology by light microscopy (upper row) and rhodamin B staining (lower row) showed compact holoclones consisting of small tightly packed cells in MCDB151 (A), spacious holoclones consisting of large flattened cells in DMEM/F12 (C), and rather irregular colonies consisting of pleomorphic cells in PCT (D) and D-KSFM (E). (F,G) Quantitative analysis of colony density (F) and colony diameter (G) showed significantly increased clonal growth in DMEM/F12 compared to MCDB151. Values represent means ± SD of five separate experiments (*$p < 0.05$; Mann-Whitney-Test).

Addition of 10% FCS and 5 ng/ml EGF to the culture medium resulted in a significantly increased colony density and size when compared to lower or higher concentrations of serum and growth factor (Fig. 6 A-D). Formation of holoclones was largely inhibited in serum-free medium, but addition of growth factors resulted in the formation of small rosette-like cell clusters, amenable to quantitative analysis. Comparison of EGF with other growth factors under serum-free culture conditions showed, that both TGF-α and KGF comparably stimulated clonal growth, whereas all other growth factors tested were significantly less effective (Fig. 6 E). Supplementation with neurotrophic factors had no effect on clonal growth, but ß-NGF showed an additive effect with EGF resulting in a 3-fold increased growth rate compared to EGF alone (Fig. 6F).

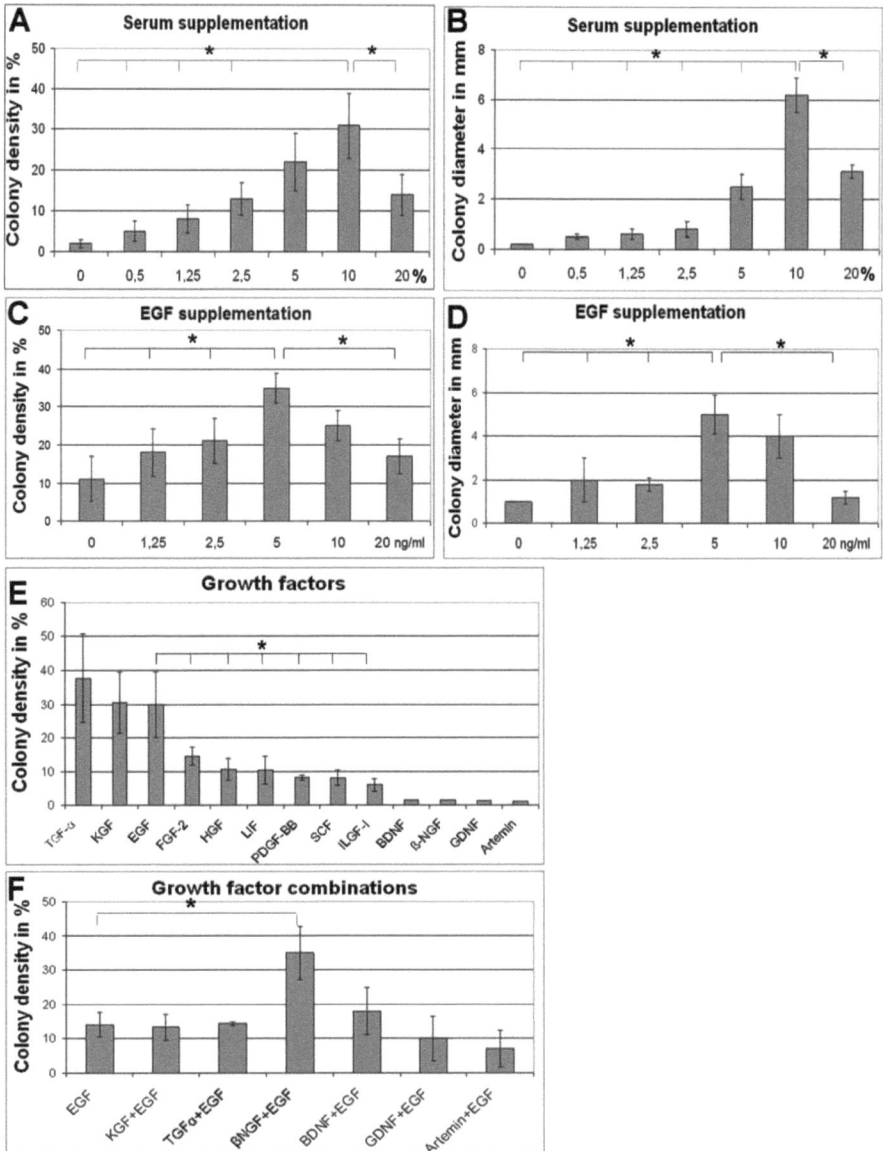

Figure 6. Effect of serum and growth factor supplementation on clonal growth.
(A,B) Quantitative analysis of colony density **(A)** and colony size **(B)** of epithelial cells cultured on a 3T3 feeder layer in MCDB151 supplemented with different concentrations of fetal calf serum (FCS) showed that addition of 10% FCS resulted in a significantly higher clonal growth rate compared to lower or higher FCS

concentrations. **(C,D)** Cultivation in serum-free MCDB151 supplemented with different concentrations of human epidermal growth factor (EGF) showed that addition of 5 ng/ml EGF resulted in a significantly higher colony density **(C)** and size **(D)** compared to lower or higher growth factor concentrations. **(E-F)** Comparative analysis of different growth factors (EGF, keratinocyte growth factor KGF, transforming growth factor-α TGF-α, platelet-derived growth factor-BB PDGF-BB, leukemia-inhibitory factor LIF, hepatocyte growth factor HGF, stem-cell factor SCF, insulin-like growth factor-I IGF-I, and fibroblast growth factor-2 FGF-2) under serum-free conditions showed that EGF, TGF-α, and KGF equally stimulated clonal growth **(E)**, whereas all other growth factors tested were significantly less effective. Supplementation with neurotrophic factors (brain-derived neurotrophic factor BDNF, nerve growth factor β-NGF, glial cell-derived neurotrophic factor GDNF and artemin) had no effect on clonal growth, but ß-NGF showed an additive effect with EGF resulting in a 3-fold increased growth rate compared to EGF alone **(F)**. Values represent means ± SD of five separate experiments (*p < 0.05; Mann-Whitney-Test).

4.1.5. Effect of culture conditions on clonal cell phenotype

Since extracellular calcium concentration is a decisive factor modulating epithelial growth and differentiation [44, 45], we compared the effect of culture media with particularly low (MCDB151) and high (DMEM/F12) calcium concentrations on the cellular phenotype. Cells in MCDB151-cultured clones were uniformly smaller and expressed less K3/K12 but higher levels of progenitor cell markers, such as ABCG2 and K15, when compared to cells cultured in DMEM/F12 medium (Fig. 7A-D). P63α as a SC determinant in holoclones [6, 42] was markedly expressed under low calcium conditions but considerably declined under high calcium conditions (Fig. 7 E,F).

Transmission electron micrographs of vertical sections through DMEM/F12-cultured colonies revealed a stratified epithelial layer composed of elongated, largely differentiated cells containing apical microvilli, prominent cytoplasmic filaments, and abundant desmosomes in all layers. In contrast, colonies grown in MCDB151 showed a basal layer of small, rather undifferentiated cuboid cells centrally covered by one to two layers of elongated cells with beginning signs of differentiation (Fig. 7 G,H).

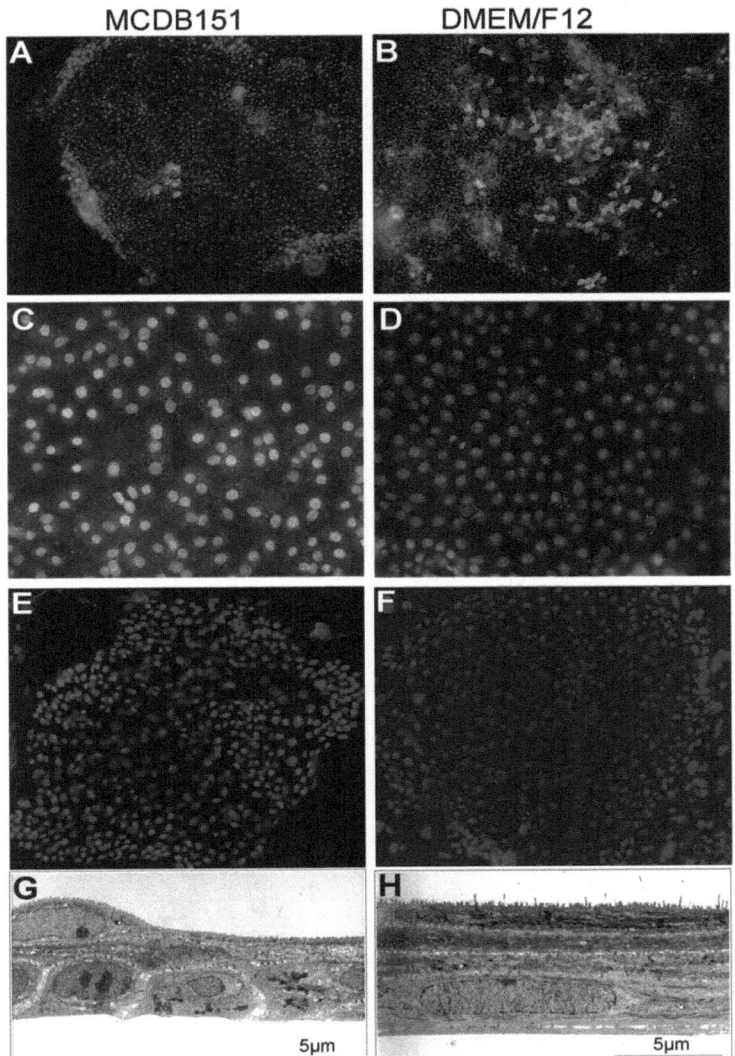

Figure 7. Effect of extracellular calcium concentration on clonal cell phenotype

(A-F) Comparative immunofluorescence analysis of holoclones expanded in culture medium with particularly low (MCDB151) and high (DMEM/F12) calcium concentrations using antibodies against stem cell (ABCG2, p63α) and differentiation (K3/K12) markers. Cells in MCDB151-cultured clones expressed lower levels of K3/K12 (A) but higher levels of ABCG2 (C) and p63α (E) when compared to cells cultured in DMEM/F12 medium (B,D,F). (G,H) Transmission electron micrographs of vertical sections through holoclones expanded in MCDB151 revealed a basal layer of small, rather undifferentiated cuboid cells covered by one to two layers of elongated cells **(G)**, whereas holoclones grown in DMEM/F12 showed a stratified epithelial layer composed of elongated, flattened and largely differentiated cells **(H)**. Nuclear staining was performed with propidium iodide (red, **A-D**) or DAPI (4´,6-diamidino-2-phenylindole) (blue, **E** and **F**). Magnification: 100x **(C,D)**, 40x **(E,F)**, 20x **(A,B)**. Scale bars = 5µm **(G,H)**

4.1.6. Generation of epithelial cell sheets on fibrin

After dissociating and transferring holoclones before adjacent colonies merged, i.e. 21 days on average, clonally expanded limbal progenitor cells were seeded onto fibrin gels. Subcultivation of cells in MCDB151 medium supplemented with 10% FCS and 5 ng/ml EGF, which was switched from low calcium (0.03 mmol/L) to medium-level calcium (0.4 mmol/L) concentrations after 7 days, gave rise to stratified cohesive epithelial cell sheets consisting of a basal layer formed by cuboid cells and 2 to 3 suprabasal layers of elongated cells, after 14-16 days in submersion culture (Fig. 8 A,C). Moderate K3/K12 expression was restricted to superficial cell layers (Fig. 8E), whereas positive staining for p63α, Bmi-1, ABCG2, and K15 was restricted to clusters of mainly basally located cells (Fig. 8G,I,K) indicating preservation of the SC phenotype within the epithelial construct. Following dissociation of cells from the fibrin substrate, CFE was calculated as 0.15%. Elevation of calcium concentration to 1.2 mmol/L produced a stratified epithelial sheet composed of 5 to 6 layers of elongated, largely differentiated cells (Fig. 8B,D). Consistently, these culture conditions caused a pronounced increase in K3/K12 expression (Fig. 8F) and a marked decline in expression of p63α, Bmi-1 and K15 (Fig. 8H,J,L). Cells detached from the fibrin gels did not retain the potential to form holoclones.

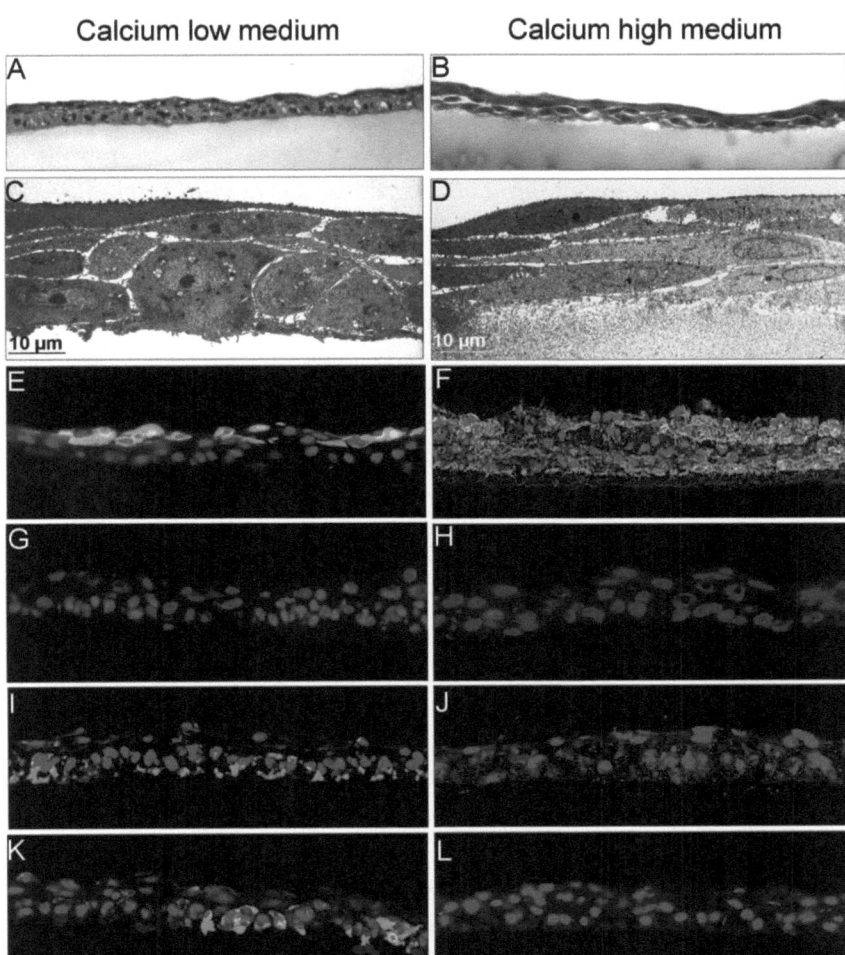

Figure 8. Generation of epithelial cell sheets on fibrin gel.

(A-L): Comparative phenotypic analysis of clonally expanded epithelial cells subcultivated on fibrin in media containing low to medium (MCDB151) or high (DMEM/F12) calcium concentrations for 14-16 days in submersion culture. **(A-D)** Light microscopic **(A,B)** and electron microscopic **(C,D)** analysis showed multilayered epithelial cell sheets consisting of a basal layer formed by cuboid cells and 2 to 3 suprabasal layers of elongated cells in MCDB151 **(A,C)**, but a stratified epithelial sheet composed of 5 to 6 layers of elongated, largely differentiated cells in DMEM/F12 **(B,D)**. Immunofluorescence analysis **(E-L)** showed that K3/K12 expression was restricted to superficial cell layers **(E)**, whereas positive staining for p63α **(G)**, Bmi-1 **(I)**, and K15 **(K)** was observed in clusters of mainly basally located cells, when MCDB151 was used as culture medium. In contrast, cultivation in DMEM/F12 caused a pronounced increase in K3/K12 expression

(F) and a marked decline in expression of p63α (H), Bmi-1 (J), and K15 (L). Staining: periodic acid-Schiff (A), hematoxylin-eosin (B). Nuclear staining was performed with propidium iodide (red, E and F, I-L) or DAPI (4´,6-diamidino-2-phenylindole) (blue, G and H). Magnification: 100x (E-L), 40x (A,B); Scale bars = 10μm (C,D).

4.2. Alternative autologous stem cell sources: murine and human hair follicles

The isolation, cultivation, phenotypic characterization and transdifferentiation experiments were initially performed on murine vibrissae-derived hair follicles (HF) because of their easier accessibility than human scalp biopsies. After having proved the general capacity of murine HF epithelial SC to trandifferentiate into corneal epithelial-like cells under appropriate culture condition, the experimental approaches were also applied with human HF SC in view of future therapeutic applications in the clinical setting.

4.2.1. Comparative expression of stem cell and differentiation markers in hair follicles and cornea

Expression patterns of putative SC and differentiation markers were compared by immunohistochemistry on frozen sections of murine hair follicle (HF) and cornea. The putative SC markers K15 and α6 integrin, which have been previously reported to be expressed in the murine HF bulge region at high levels [46, 47], were confirmed to be strongly expressed in both bulge cells and basal cells of the HF outer root sheath (Fig. 9A,B,D,E). Whereas K15 could be immunolocalized to the cytoplasm of bulge and basal cells (Fig. 9A,B), α6 integrin was more widely expressed and localized to cell membranes of bulge and basal cells (Fig. 9D,E). Both markers were also observed in the murine corneo-limbal region showing distinct K15 staining of basal cells in the limbal epithelium (Fig. 9C) and α6 integrin staining of basal cells in the corneal epithelium (Fig. 9F). K10, a marker of terminally differentiated epidermal keratinocytes, was neither expressed in HF nor corneal epithelial cells (data not shown). K12, a marker of differentiated corneal epithelial cells, was found to be expressed exclusively in the corneal epithelium (Fig. 9H) but not in the HF (Fig. 9G). Pax6, a transcription factor for K12, was found to be expressed mainly in the basal cells of the corneal epithelium (Fig.9I) but was also lacking in the HF (Fig. 9G). A similar expression pattern of SC and differentiation markers was observed in human HF and corneo-limbal region (data not shown). These different expression patterns in HF and cornea were confirmed using real-time RT-PCR and Western blotting (data not shown). Together, these observations indicate important parallels regarding SC markers and differences regarding differentiation markers between the HF and the corneo-limbal region in both mouse and human model.

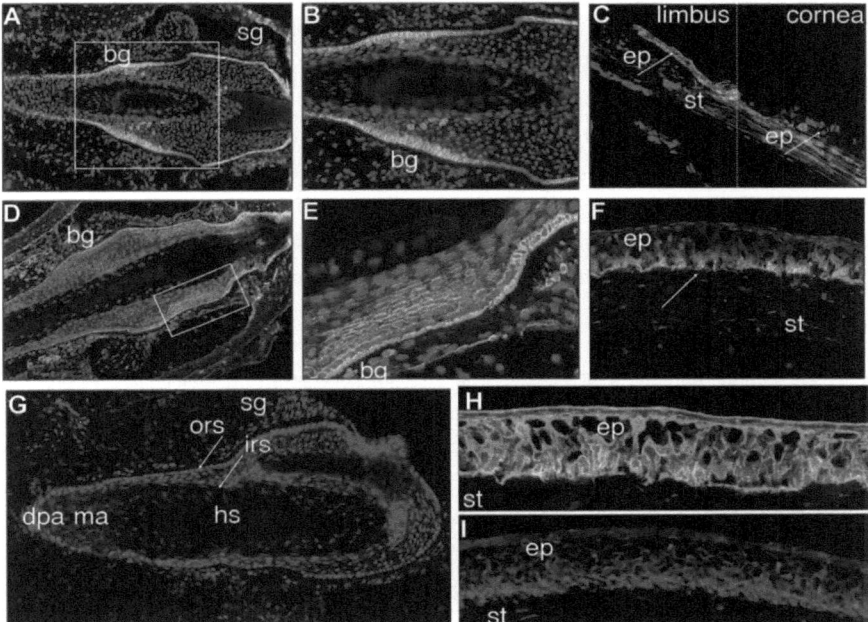

Figure 9. Expression of stem cell and differentiation markers in murine hair follicle (HF) and cornea. (A,B): Expression of K15, a putative epithelial stem and progenitor cell marker, in the HF bulge and basal cells. (C): Selective expression of K15 in the basal cells of limbal epithelium. (D,E): Expression of α6 integrin, a putative stem and progenitor cell marker, in HF bulge and basal cells. (F): Expression of α6 integrin in the basal cells of the corneal epithelium. (G): Lack of expression of K12 and Pax6 in the murine vibrissae HF. (H): Expression of K12 (green fluorescence) in murine corneal epithelium. (I): Expression of Pax6 (red fluorescence) in the cell nuclei of corneal epithelium throughout all the epithelial cell layers. Nuclear staining was performed with propidium iodide (red) or DAPI (blue). Magnification: x 200 (E,I,H), x 100 (B,C,F,G), x 40 (A,D). Abbreviations: bg, bulge; dpa, dermal papilla; ep, epithelium; hs, hair shaft; irs, inner rooth sheath; ma, matrix; ors, outer root sheath; sg, sebaceous gland; st, stroma

4.2.2. Isolation and clonal enrichment of murine and human hair follicle bulge cells

To isolate HF bulge cells and to enrich colony forming epithelial SC, two different approaches were performed and compared regarding colony forming efficiency (CFE) and phenotype of clonal cells: (1) mechanical dissection and enzymatic dissociation of the murine and human bulge cells and (2)

fluorescence-activated cell sorting (FACS) of murine HF cells using an antibody against α6 integrin.

For mechanical separation and enzymatic digestion, either murine vibrissae HF or human scalp HF (n=50), measuring on average 3 mm or 5 mm in length, respectively, and comprising the epithelial root sheaths, the bulge, the sebaceous gland, and the dermal papilla (Fig. 10A), were dissected and carefully cut into three fragments (Fig. 10B). The section containing the sebaceous gland was designated as S1, the bulge-containing section was designated S2, and the remaining part containing matrix and papilla was indicated S3. To evaluate the clonogenic potential of the different portions, single cell suspensions obtained from each section were plated onto a 3T3 feeder layer, cultivated for 14 days in calcium-low (0.4 mM Ca2+) medium, and then fixed and stained with 2% rhodamine B. Whereas cells isolated from regions S1 and S3 were not clonogenic, only cells isolated from the bulge region S2 gave rise to large colonies measuring up to 10 mm in diameter with smooth perimeters, termed holoclones [27] (Fig. 10C). The CFE, which is considered to correlate with the number of SC present in the S2 cell population, was calculated to be 0.1% by murine (Fig. 10G) and 0.15% by human bulge SC. Clonal cells could be serially cultivated up to 6 passages before they revealed phenotypic signs of senescence. These observations confirm previous reports, that clonogenic cells with high proliferative capacity, a typical characteristic of SC, are segregated in the bulge region of the murine and human HF [48]. Consistently, murine explant cultures revealed cellular outgrowth and colony formation from the bulge region after 7-10 days (Fig. 11A). The outgrowing cells were immunopositive for the putative stem cell marker K15 (Fig. 11B).

In a second approach, freshly isolated murine HF cells were sorted by FACS using a FITC-conjugated antibody against α6 integrin (Fig. 10D). The resulting populations of α6-positive cells, representing about 5% of the total cell population, and α6-negative cells were seeded at a definite clonal density on a 3T3 feeder layer. After two weeks of culture, keratinocyte colonies were compared regarding CFE and immunopositivity for α6 integrin. The α6-positive cell population exhibited a significantly higher clonogenic capacity with formation of holoclones compared with the α6-negative cell population producing few paraclones only (Fig. 10E,F). The CFE of the α6-positive cell population was calculated to be 0.3% (Fig. 10G).

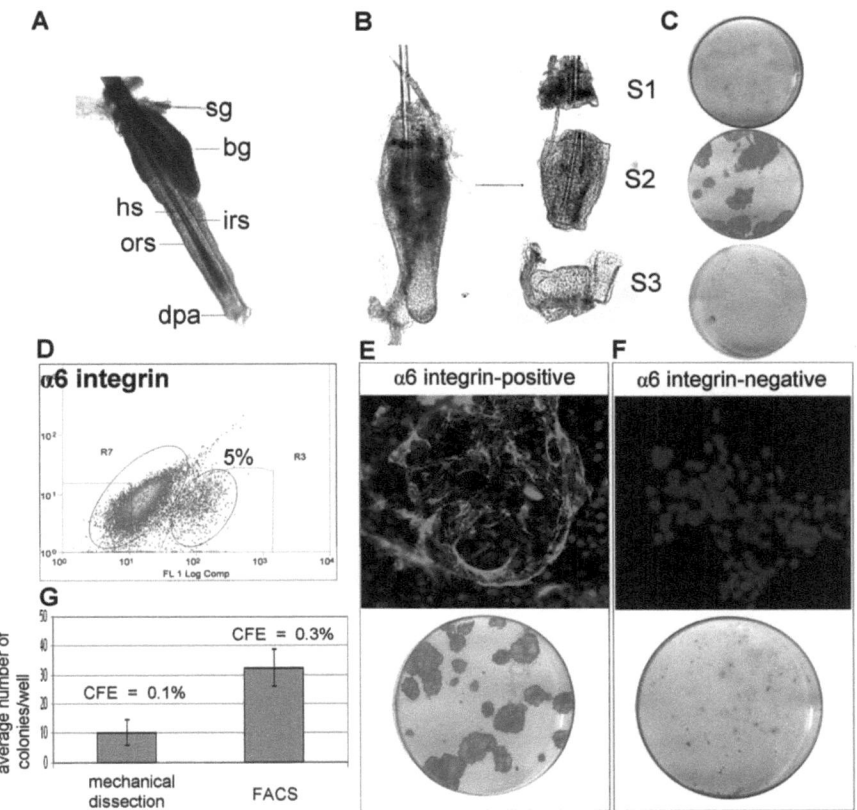

Figure 10. Isolation of hair follicle (HF) bulge cells. (A): Isolated HF after enzymatic digestion of the collagen capsule. **(B):** Dissection of the isolated HF into 3 fragments: (S1) sebaceous gland containing section, (S2) bulge containing section and (S3) dermal papilla and matrix containing section. **(C):** Colony forming assay performed with cells derived from S1, S2 and S3 on a 3T3 feeder cell layer, rhodamin B staining after 2 weeks of culture. **(D):** Fluorescence-activated cell sorting (FACS) of isolated HF cells using an antibody to α6 integrin; the α6 integrin-positive cell population accounts for about 5% of total cells. **(E):** Clonogenic capacity of α6 integrin-positive **(F):** and α6 integrin-negative cell populations obtained by FACS. **(G):** Calculation of the colony-forming efficiency (CFE) of a α6 integrin-positive cell population after cell sorting in comparison to CFE of the bulge cells after mechanical dissection. The bar chart demonstrates the mean number of colonies ± SD from 5 experiments. Magnification: x 100 **(E,F)**, x 40 **(A,B)**. Abbreviations: bg, bulge; dpa, dermal papilla; hs, hair shaft; irs, inner root sheath; ors, outer root sheath; sg, sebaceous gland.

Phenotypic characterization of holoclones formed by either mechanical dissection or FACS showed their composition of small, roundish, densely packed cells independent of the method of cell isolation (Fig. 11C). By immunocytochemistry, a few K15-positive cells, supposed to represent

Results

putative stem or progenitor cells, were present in the center of murine (Fig. 11D) and rather close to the perimeter in human holoclones. Most holoclones revealed a central focus of stratification with suprabasal cells expressing K10 typical of epidermal differentiation (Fig. 11E). The cornea-specific marker K12 was not expressed within the colonies (Fig. 11F). The proportion of K10-positive cells within the holoclones could be increased by elevating the calcium concentration (1.2 mM Ca2+) of the culture medium (data not shown).

These findings indicate that both mechanical dissection and FACS using α6 integrin antibodies followed by clonal expansion are effective methods to isolate and enrich epithelial stem and progenitor cell populations from the murine and human HF bulge region.

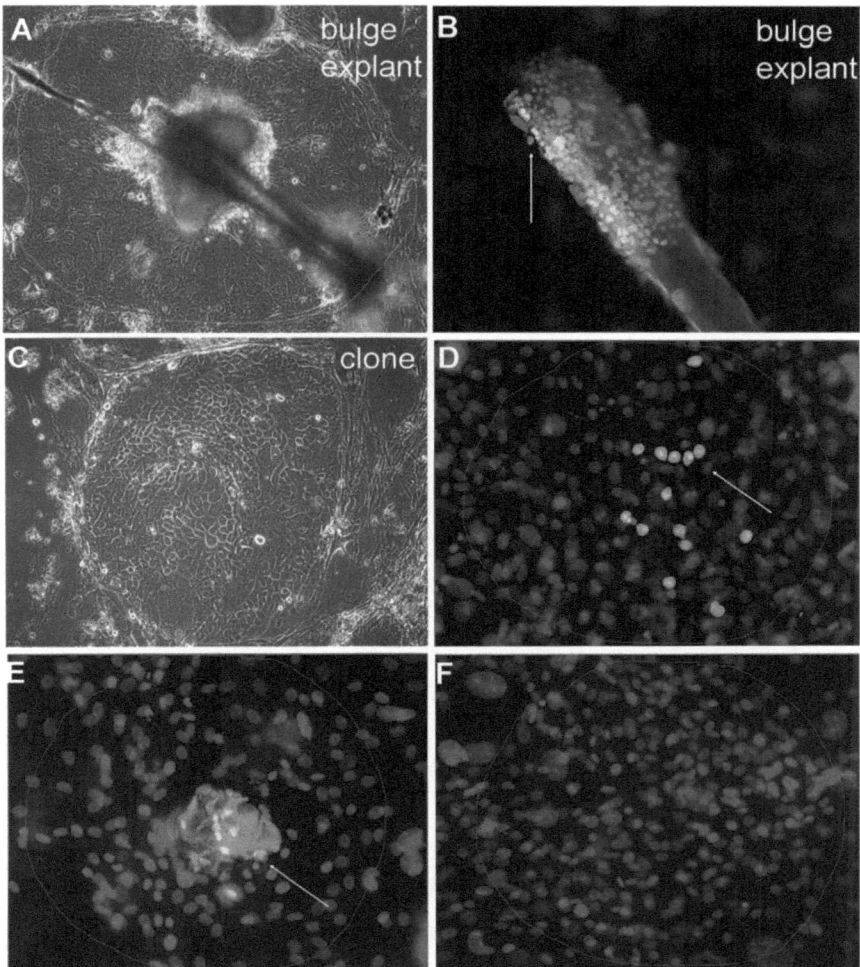

Figure 11. Clonal enrichment of hair follicle (HF) bulge cells. (A): Cellular outgrowth of HF bulge explants after 7-10 days of culture on a 3T3 feeder layer. (B): Expression of K15, an epithelial stem cell marker, in the outgrowing cells (arrow) of a bulge tissue explant. (C): Light microscopy of a holoclone obtained by either mechanical dissection or fluorescence-activated cell sorting on a 3T3 feeder layer. (D): K15-positive basal cells (arrow) are present in the culture of a holoclone. (E): K10-positive cells (arrow) are present in the culture of a holoclone, confined to a suprabasal layer of the central focus of stratification. (F): Lack of K12 expression within a holoclone. Nuclear staining was performed with propidium iodide (red). Magnification: x 100 (D, E,F), x 40 (A,B,C)

4.2.3. Effect of environmental conditions on growth and differentiation of murine and human hair follicle stem cells

Previous studies implicated type IV collagen, laminin-1, laminin-5, and fibronectin as major components of the basement membrane zone of corneal and limbal epithelia [9]. Murine clonal cells subcultivated on these matrix components showed significant differences in their adhesion properties. Subcultivation on type IV collagen and laminin-5 resulted in rapid cell adhesion and growth with about 90% of murine cells becoming adherent within 30 minutes after seeding. Both matrices supported the formation of regularly arranged monolayers of cuboid cells in a comparable manner (Fig. 12A,C). In contrast, laminin-1, fibronectin as well as uncoated culture plates adversely affected murine cell adhesion and growth resulting in about 10% of cells becoming attached to the substrates without formation of a confluent monolayer (Fig. 12B,D).

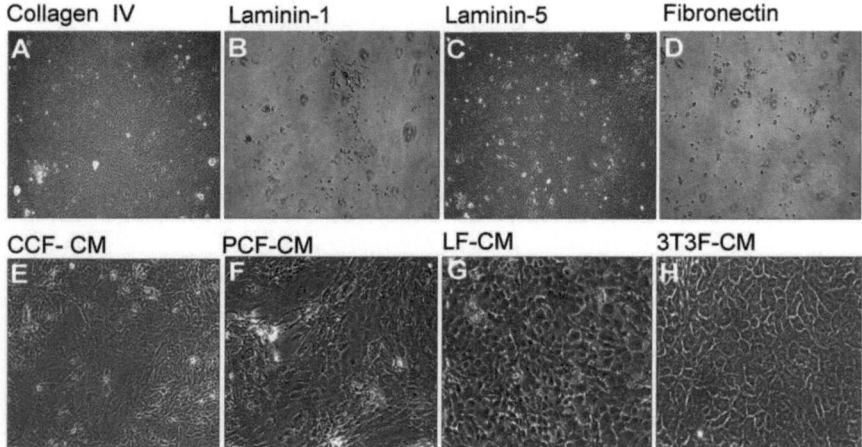

Figure 12. Effect of various culture conditions (matrices and conditioned media) on growth of clonally enriched, subcultivated hair follicle stem cells. (A-D): Light microscopic appearance of clonal cells subcultivated on **(A):** type IV collagen, **(B):** laminin-1, **(C):** laminin-5, and **(D):** fibronectin. **(A,C):** Cultivation on type IV collagen and laminin-5 resulted in formation of regular epitheloid cell layers, whereas **(B,D):** laminin-1 and fibronectin adversely affected cell adhesion and growth. **(E-H):** Light microscopic appearance of clonal cells subcultivated on laminin-5 in various CM from **(E):** central corneal fibroblasts (CCF-CM), **(F):** peripheral corneal fibroblasts (PCF-CM), **(G):** limbal fibroblasts (LF-CM), and **(H):** 3T3 fibroblasts (3T3F-CM). **(G,H):** LF-CM and 3T3F-CM induced formation of regularly arranged, epitheloid cell sheets, whereas **(E,F):** CCF-CM and PCF-CM resulted in rather irregular growth patterns of cells. Magnification: x 100 **(A-D)**, x 200 **(E-H)**.

Results

For further experiments, laminin-5 was selected as a substrate, because it represents a more specific component of the corneo-limbal basement membrane zone than the rather ubiquitous basement membrane component type IV collagen. Murine clonal cells subcultivated on laminin-5 in various conditioned media for 7 days in calcium-medium and then about 7 days in calcium-high (1.2 mM Ca^{2+}) conditions showed significant differences in their growth patterns. Subcultivation in CM obtained from central and peripheral corneal fibroblasts resulted in rather irregular growth patterns revealing partly enlarged and flattened, and partly elongated cells (Fig. 12E,F). Using CM from limbal fibroblasts, clonal cells formed confluent, regularly arranged, cobble stone-like cell sheets composed of small cuboid cells (Fig. 12G), similar to cells grown in CM from 3T3 fibroblasts (Fig. 12H).

The effect of different CM on K10 and K12 protein expression was analyzed by immunohistochemistry of murine clonal cells subcultivated in laminin-5 coated chamber slides. As expected, both markers could be immunolocalized to cytoplasmic filaments, but the proportion of K10- and K12-immunopositive cells showed significant differences depending on the CM used. As compared to 3T3 CM, CM obtained from central and peripheral corneal fibroblasts produced markedly higher proportions of K10-positive cells, whereas CM derived from limbal fibroblasts produced only few K10-positive cells (Fig. 13A-D). In contrast, K12 protein expression was most pronounced in cells subcultivated in limbal CM, but markedly weaker in both corneal CM and in 3T3 CM (Fig. 13E-H).

To verify the immunocytochemical findings, murine mRNA and protein expression of K10, K12, and additionally transcription factor Pax6, in response to different CM were analyzed by real time RT-PCR and Western blotting. Consistently, K10 mRNA expression was reduced in limbal CM (about 5-fold; $p<0.05$) and increased in both corneal CM compared with 3T3 CM (Fig. 13I). In contrast, K12 mRNA expression level was significantly increased in limbal CM (about 5-fold; $p<0.005$) compared with the other CM derived from corneal and 3T3 fibroblasts (Fig. 13J). Concordantly, Pax6 expression was most pronounced in limbal CM, while it was hardly detectable in 3T3 CM (Fig. 13K). Western blot analysis confirmed the highest expression levels of K12 and Pax6 protein in cells cultivated in limbal CM, whereas K10 protein expression was lowest under these conditions (Fig. 13L,M). 3T3 CM was found to suppress expression of both K12 and Pax6, but to induce expression of K10 (Fig. 13L,M).

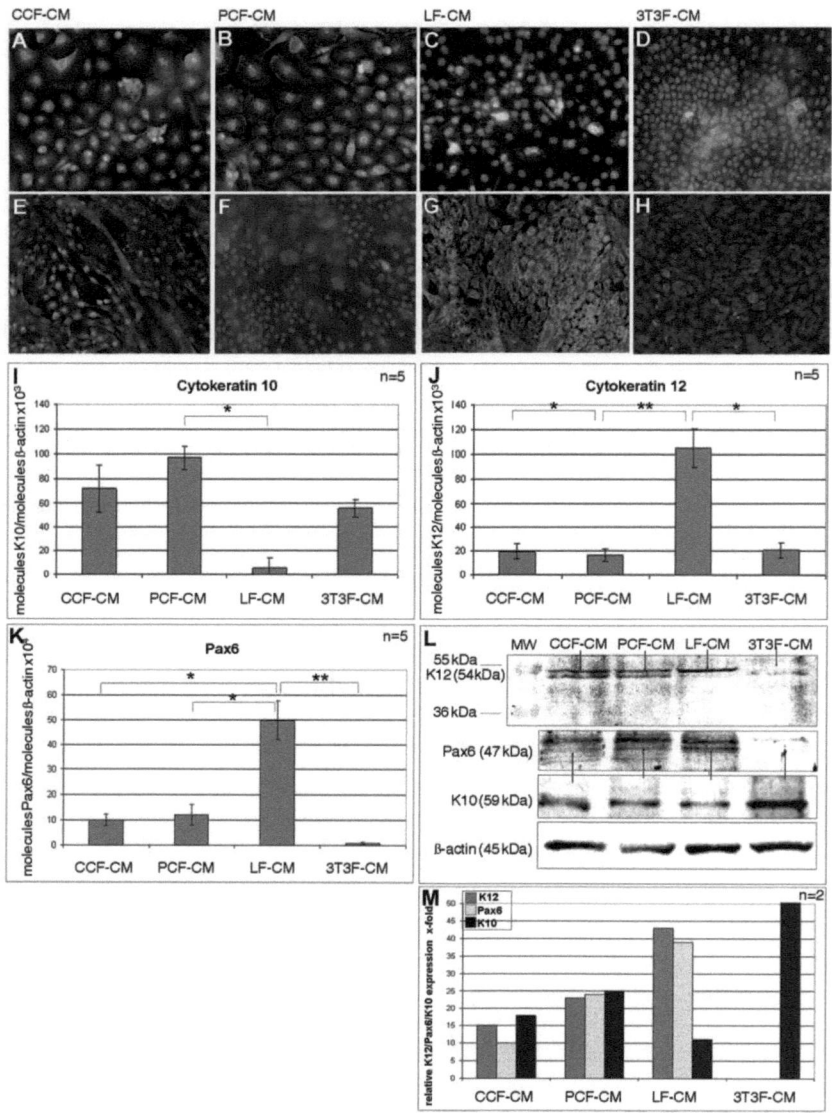

Figure 13. Effect of various conditioned media on differentiation of clonally enriched hair follicle stem cells subcultivated on laminin-5. (A-D): Expression of K10, an epidermal differentiation marker, in clonal cells exposed to conditioned medium (CM) from (A): central corneal fibroblasts (CCF-CM), (B): peripheral corneal fibroblasts (PCF-CM), (C): limbal fibroblasts (LF-CM) and, (D): 3T3 fibroblasts (3T3F-CM).

(E-H): Expression of K12, a corneal differentiation marker, in clonal cells exposed to CM from (E): central corneal fibroblasts (CCF-CM), (F): peripheral corneal fibroblasts (PCF-CM), (G): limbal fibroblasts (LF-CM) and, (H): 3T3 fibroblasts (3T3F-CM). Lowest expression of K10 (C) and highest expression of K12 (G) was observed in cells cultured in LF-CM. Nuclear staining was performed with propidium iodide (red) or DAPI (blue). Magnification: x 100. (I-K): Quantitative determination of K10, K12 and Pax6 mRNA expression levels of clonal cells cultured in various CM using real time RT-PCR technology. The expression level was normalized against β-actin expression. Lowest expression of K10 (I) and highest expression of K12 (J) and Pax6 (K) were observed in cells cultured in LF-CM. Statistical significance was assessed using the Mann-Whitney-Test for non-parametric analysis (*, $p < 0.05$, **, $p < 0.005$). (L,M): Determination of K12, K10, and Pax6 protein levels in cells cultured in different CM by Western blot analysis based on β-actin loading control. (L): Representative Western blot of cells cultured in CM from central corneal fibroblasts (CCF-CM), peripheral corneal fibroblasts (PCF-CM), limbal fibroblasts (LF-CM) and, 3T3 fibroblasts (3T3F-CM); MW, molecular weight marker. (M): Densitometric analysis of specific immunoreactive bands. Data were normalized to β-actin and represent the mean of two independent experiments.

Human HF bulge SC were cultivated in uncoated culture plates because they showed no differences in adhesion to different matrix components (type IV collagene, laminin-1, laminin-5, fibronectin) as compared to uncoated dishes. However, cultivation of human HF bulge cells in different calf-derived CM resulted in a differential expression pattern of tissue-specific markers. Consistent with the results obtained from the murine experiments, K10 mRNA expression was significantly reduced (about 20-fold; $p< 0.05$) in all CM tested compared to the unconditioned control and corresponding to expression levels in limbal SC clones (Fig. 14A). In contrast, K12 and Pax6 expression after cultivation in limbal CM was significantly elevated (15- and 20-fold, respectively) as compared to the unconditioned control and corresponding to expression levels of limbal SC clones, too (Fig.14B). Protein expression data gained by means of Western blot analyses were consistent with the real time RT-PCR data on mRNA level confirming the induction of K12 expression and reduction of K10 expression during cultivation in limbal CM (Fig. 14C).

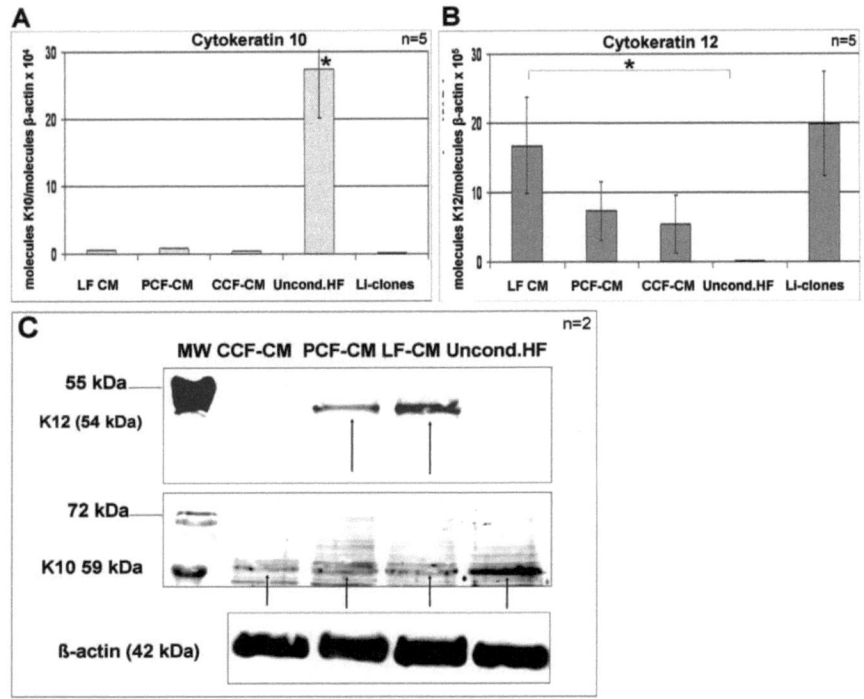

Figure 14. Effect of various conditioned media on differentiation of clonally enriched, subcultivated human hair follicle stem cells. Qantitative determination of K10 and K12 mRNA expression levels of clonal cells cultured in the following conditioned media (CM): central corneal fibroblasts (CCF-CM), peripheral corneal fibroblasts (PCF-CM), limbal fibroblasts (LF-CM), and using real time RT-PCR technology. Hair follicle clonal cells (uncond.HF) and limbal clonal cells (Li-clones) cultured in unconditioned medium served as controls. The expression levels were normalized against β-actin expression. **(A):** K10 mRNA expression was significantly reduced (about 20-fold) in all CM tested compared to the unconditioned control and corresponding to expression levels of limbal SC clones. **(B):** Elevated expression of K12 (about 10-fold) was observed in LF-CM compared to hair follicle cells cultured in unconditioned medium. Statistical significance was assessed using the Mann-Whitney-Test for non-parametric analysis (*, $p < 0.05$). **(C):** Determination of K10 and K12 protein levels in cells cultured in different CM by Western blot analysis based on β-actin loading control. Representative Western blot of human hair follicle cells cultured in CM from central corneal fibroblasts (CCF-CM), peripheral corneal fibroblasts (PCF-CM), limbal fibroblasts (LF-CM) and in unconditioned medium (uncond.HF); MW, molecular weight marker.

For light and electron microscopic analysis of cell sheets, murine clonal cells were subcultivated on fibrin gels coated with laminin-5 in different CM. By light microscopy, both limbal and 3T3 CM were confirmed to produce regular cell sheets composed of small epitheloid cells arranged in one or two layers after 8 to 10 days (Fig. 15A) and three to five layers after 14 to 16 days of culture (Fig. 15B). Transmission electron microscopy revealed cuboid to elongated cells containing euchromatin-rich nuclei with prominent nucleoli and showing ultrastructural signs of epithelial differentiation, such as apical microvilli, keratin filaments, hemidesmosomes, and desmosomes between adjacent cells, already apparent after one week of culture (Fig. 15C,E) and more pronounced after a prolonged culture time (Fig. 15D,F).

Immunohistological analysis revealed that stratified murine epithelial cell sheets cultured in CM from limbal fibroblasts expressed α6 integrin in all cells and K15 in single cells of the basal cell layer (Fig. 15G,H) indicating preservation of stem and progenitor cells in culture. Weak expression of K10 was confined to the superficial cell layer (Fig. 15I), whereas K12 expression was more prominent throughout all epithelial cell layers (Fig. 15J). The transcription factor Pax6 was immunolocalized to nuclei of most epithelial cells throughout all cell layers (Fig. 15K) and co-localized with K12 (Fig. 15L).

Consistently, immunochistochemical analysis of human fibrin-based HF constructs cultured in limbal CM for two weeks showed a comparable SC- and differentiation pattern of marker expression (data not shown).

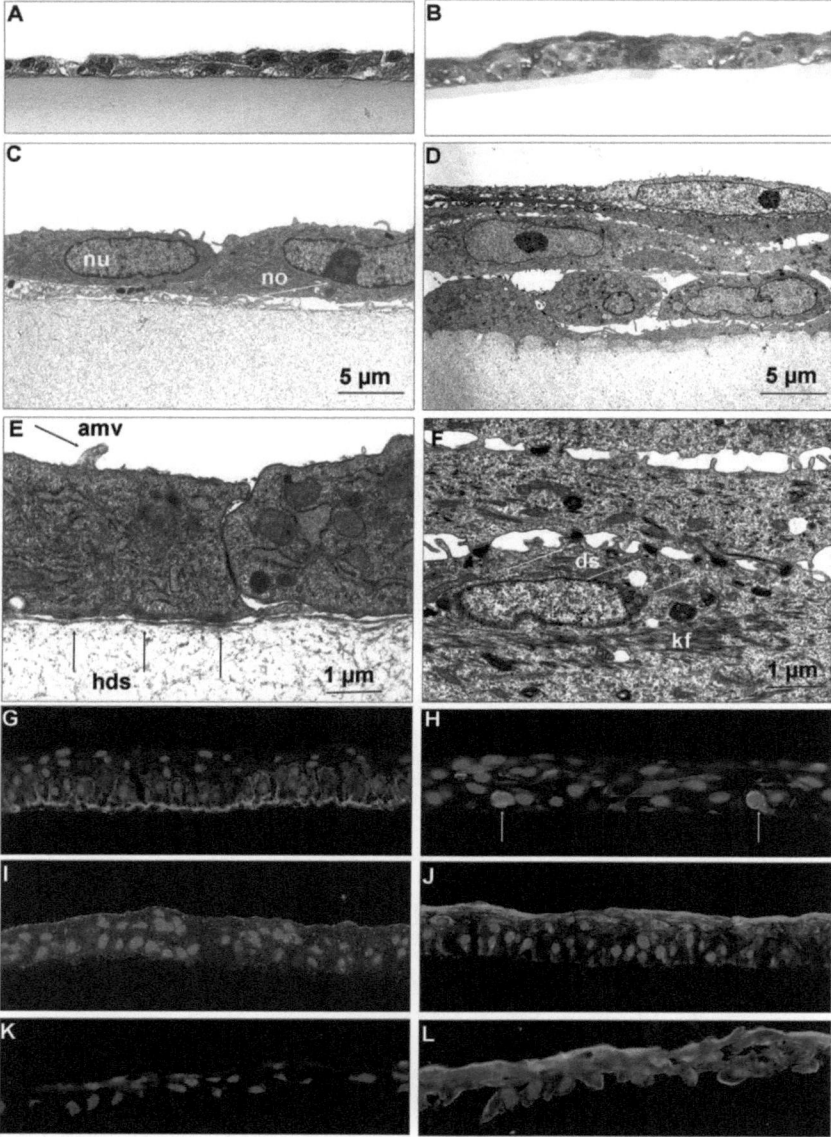

Figure 15. Phenotypic appearance of cell sheets subcultivated in limbal fibroblast conditioned medium on fibrin gels coated with laminin-5. (A,C,E): Light and electron microscopic appearance of a two-layered epithelial cell sheet after one week of culture. **(B,D,F):** Light and electron microscopic appearance of a multi-layered cell sheet after two weeks of culture. The cells show ultrastructural signs of

epithelial differentiation such as apical microvilli, keratin filaments, desmosomes and hemidesmosome. **(G):** Expression of α6 integrin (green fluorescence), a putative stem and progenitor cell marker, in the basal cell layer of epithelial sheet. **(H):** Expression of K15 (green fluorescence), a putative stem cell marker, in few single basal cells of epithelial sheet (arrows). **(I):** Expression of K10 (green fluorescence), a marker of epidermal differentiation, in the superficial cell layer. **(J):** Expression of K12 (green fluorescence), a marker of corneal differentiation, throughout all epithelial cell layers**. (K):** Expression of Pax6 (red fluorescence), a transcription factor for K12, in nuclei of epithelial cells. **(L):** Co-localization of K12 (green) and Pax6 (red) expression in epithelial cells. Staining: hematoxylin-eosin **(A)**, periodic acid-Schiff **(B)**. Magnification: x 100 **(B,G,I,K,J)**, x 200 **(A,H,L)**. Scale bars = 5 µm **(C,D)**, and 1 µm **(E,F)**. Nuclear staining was performed with propidium iodide (red) or DAPI (blue). Abbreviation: amv, apical microvilli; ds, desmosomes; hds, hemidesmosomes; kf, keratin filaments; no, nucleolus; nu, nucleus

Collectively, this data indicate that the phenotype and differentiation of HF epithelial SC can be influenced by a specific microenvironment and that factors derived from limbal fibroblasts appear to induce expression of the corneal epithelial differentiation marker K12 together with its transcription factor Pax6, while factors derived from corneal fibroblasts rather promote expression of the epidermal differentiation marker K10.

4.2.4. Premilinary engraftment experiments of cultivated hair follicle epithelial sheets

As pilot experiments for further *in vivo* animal studies on the functionality of the human HF epithelial construct, a limbal stem cell deficiency (LSCD) model was created in two rabbit eyes. Healthy, untreated contralateral eyes served as control (Fig. 16A). Subcultured human HF clonal cells formed confluent epithelial sheets on the fibrin gel after 14 days of culture in limbal CM, consisting of 4 to 5 layers of stratified epithelium, with cuboidal to columnar basal cells, and progressive flattening cells toward the surface (Fig. 16 C). This cultivated HF epithelial fibrin-based construct was successfully transplanted onto the damaged cornea of one rabbit eye. Complete epithelialization was confirmed by slit lamp biomicroscopy, fluorescein staining and corneal transparency until one week post engraftment (Fig. 16B). For histological analysis, the treated and untreted eyes were enucleated 7 days post engraftment. After one week the cornea was completely epithelialized and revealed multilayered epithelial sheets with small cuboid cells in the basal and suprabasal layers and flattened elongated cells in the superficial layers. There were no signs of vascularisation, inflammation and the corneal opacity was not interfered.
The HF graft stained positively for the anti-human nuclei antibody (Fig. 16D) proving evidence for the graft cells on the top of the rabbit cornea.

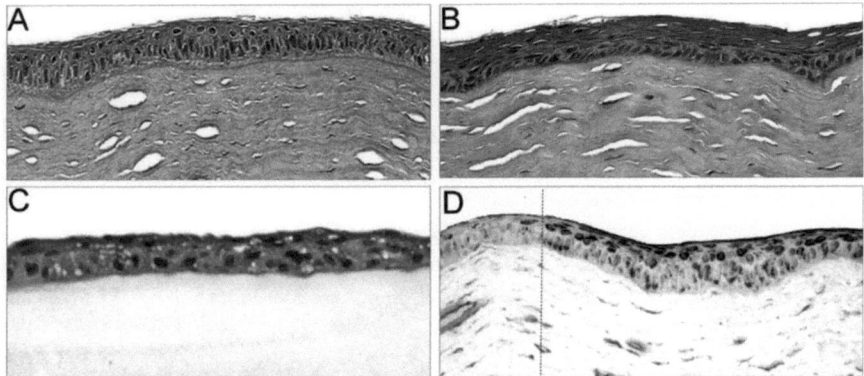

Figure 16. Light microscopic appearance of cell sheets reconstructed from human hair follicle stem cells pre- and post-engraftment onto a rabbit eye. (A): Corneal epithelium of the healthy contralateral rabbit eye. **(B):** HF-derived epithelial cell sheets reconstituting the corneal epithelium 7 days post engraftment in rabbit model with total LSCD. **(C):** HF-derived epithelial fibrin-based construct prior to engraftment. **(D):** Positive staining of the graft cells for the anti-human nuclei antibody (brown nuclear staining). The dashed line indicates the border between the human HF-derived epithelial construct and the rabbit epithelium. Staining: periodic acid-Schiff **(A-C)**. Magnification: x 40 **(A,B)**, x 100 **(C,D)**.

The engrafted cultivated HF epithelial constructs examined 7 days post engraftment revealed a moderate expression of K12, a corneal differentiation marker, throughout all the graft layers except for the basal and suprabasal layers using a specific anti-human antibody. In contrast, there was no positive staining for K12 in a control healthy rabbit corneal epithelium (Fig. 17A, left and right panel). The epidermal differentiation marker K10 was weakly expressed in the basal and suprabasal layers of the graft 7 days postoperatively, whereas there was no positive staining for K10 in the control cornea (Fig. 17B). The stem and progenitor cell marker K15 was prominently expressed in the basal layer of the graft pointing to the presence and maintenance of the immature cells within the graft up to one week post engraftment (Fig.17C). Consistently, there was no K15 expression in the control rabbit cornea confirming once again the high specificity of the anti-human antibodies and thus the human origin of the grafted HF cells.

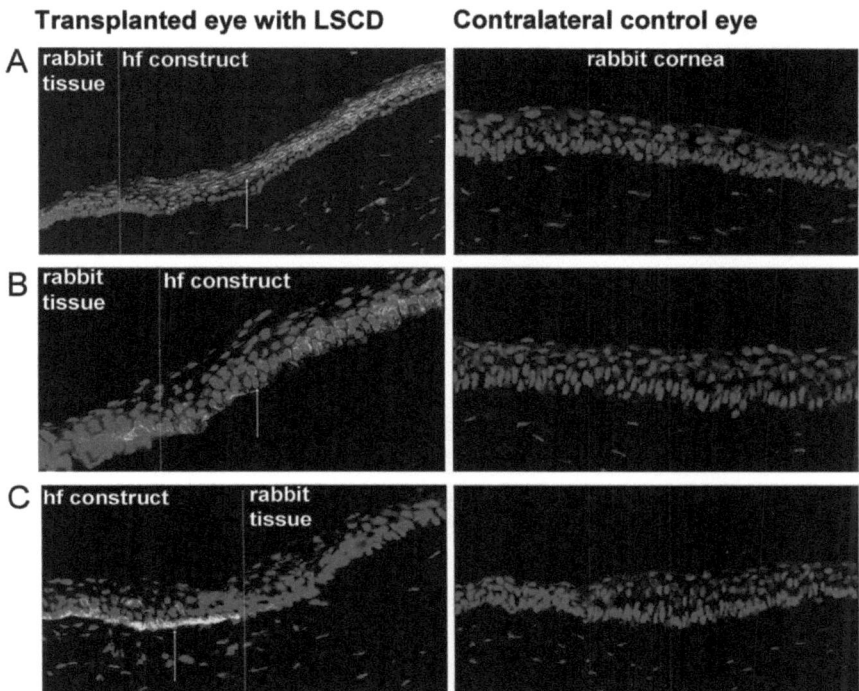

Figure 17. Immunohistochemical characterization of hair follicle-derived epithelial graft 1 week post-operatively in comparison with a healthy untreated rabbit eye (right panel). (A): Moderate expression of K12, a marker of corneal differentiation, in observed throughout all superficial layers of the graft (green staining, arrow) using a specific anti-human K12 antibody (B): Weak expression of K10, a marker of epidermal differentiation, is seen in the basal and suprabasal layers of the graft (green staining, arrow) but not in the corneal epithelium of the control eye. (C): Marked expression of K15, a stem and progenitor cell marker, in the basal layer of the graft (arrow) (left panel); no positive staining for K15 of the control rabbit cornea. Magnification: x 40 (A left panel), x 100 (B,C). Nuclear staining was performed with propidium iodide (red). Abbreviation: hf, hair follicle; LSCD, limbal stem cell deficiency.

In conclusion, these preliminary results of the engraftment experiments indicate that, HF bulge SC may represent a novel promising source of autologous adult SC for tissue engineering approaches for ocular surface reconstruction in patients with LSCD.

5. Discussion

5.1. Optimization of cell culture conditions for ex vivo expansion of limbal epithelial stem and progenitor cells

Transplantation of *ex vivo* expanded limbal epithelial cells has become a routine treatment for ocular surface reconstruction in patients with unilateral limbal LSCD in several clinical centers [19]. However, the widespread use of cultured limbal epithelial autografts has been hampered by different techniques of cultivation and variable clinical results reported. Differences in culture techniques include the use of explant or single cell suspension systems, the presence or absence of a 3T3 feeder layer, the use of different carriers including fibrin and amniotic membrane, and the use or not of airlifting to promote epithelial differentiation and stratification. The most widely used method is the explant culture system, in which a small limbal biopsy is placed on the carrier and the limbal epithelial cells then migrate out of the biopsy and proliferate to form an epithelial sheet [49-54]. However, outgrowths from human limbal explants show a rapid decline in proliferative potential and it is assumed that TAC rather than SC actually migrate onto the culture substrate [23]. Using limbal epithelial cell suspensions instead of limbal explants may increase the proportion of SC in the culture system [55-59]. Nevertheless, it is still unclear whether cultivated epithelial sheets contain sufficient amounts of limbal stem and progenitor cells, which is the key prerequisite to ensure successful and long-term regeneration of the ocular surface [60, 61].

In this work, we present an optimized method for the expansion of epithelial SC derived from a small limbal biopsy, which greatly increases the survival of stem and progenitor cells in culture. The system uses clonal enrichment of limbal SC and their subcultivation on fibrin as a transplantable carrier. It is based on Rheinwald and Green's pioneering work (1975), showing that human epidermal SC can be expanded by clonal growth on a fibroblast feeder layer, which has been later adapted to the amplification of limbal SC by Pellegrini and associates [18, 41]. Subsequently, cultivated epithelial sheets seeded with clonally enriched stem and progenitor cells have been used as epidermal autografts for long-term skin replacement [28, 31] and ocular surface reconstruction [29, 30], and demonstration of holoclones within epithelial grafts has been considered a means of quality control [6]. However, it has been stressed that improper culture conditions can irreversibly induce clonal conversion and hence cause a rapid disappearance of SC, strengthening the importance of a thorough evaluation of the impact of cultivation procedures on SC behaviour and phenotype.

In this work, we have used an analysis of colony growth, measured by CFE, colony size, and colony density, to objectively evaluate the effects of culture variables and to screen for agents

Discussion

with growth-promoting activities. The findings provide evidence that the efficacy of SC isolation is highest using biopsies from the superior limbus, which showed the greatest CFE, and a combined dispase II/trypsin-EDTA enzymatic dissociation method. It has been suggested previously that corneal SC are not evenly distributed throughout the human limbus, being more abundant in the inferior and superior regions than in the nasal and temporal regions [62-64], although others have reported on a higher CFE in the superior and temporal quadrants [41]. The precise sampling location is particularly relevant, when limited amounts of tissue are available for SC isolation and expansion. We have demonstrated here that an initial biopsy of 2 mm^2 taken from the superior limbus of a 50-year-old donor yielded approximately 2×10^4 cells and could be clonally expanded in vitro to $1-2 \times 10^6$ cells. However, the CFE declined with the age of the donor, which is in consistency with previous reports [27, 30].

Clonal growth and preservation of SC require both the presence of a 3T3 feeder layer and proper serum concentrations [25-27, 30, 41, 65, 66]. Furthermore, addition of growth factors, most importantly EGF or TGFα, to the culture medium has become a standard requisite [27, 65-68]. In this study, 10% FCS was the optimum concentration to stimulate CFE and colony growth. The clonogenic potential was further increased by addition of 5 ng/ml EGF to the medium, but equal concentrations of TGFα or KGF were found to be similarly effective in increasing the clonal growth rate. KGF is highly expressed by limbal fibroblasts suggesting that KGF might be involved in modulating limbal SC function [69]. However, cells grown in the presence of both EGF and ß-NGF showed the highest rate of colony expansion, which was increased about 3-fold compared to EGF alone. β-NGF has been associated with the proliferation and differentiation of human corneal epithelial cells [70]. Its high affinity receptor TrkA is expressed in both corneal and limbal epithelial basal cells suggesting that NGF signalling supports limbal SC survival in vivo [14]. Blocking NGF signalling significantly retarded cell expansion on amniotic membrane supporting the notion that NGF is also important for the expansion of limbal epithelial progenitor cells in vitro [71].

To support long-term preservation and proliferation of SC and their progenitors, holoclones were maintained in a growth medium (MCDB151 supplemented with hydrocortisone, insulin, and transferrin) containing extremely low calcium concentrations (0.03 mmol/L). It is well known that increasing concentrations of extracellular calcium induce epithelial cell differentiation [44, 45, 72-74]. Consistently, clonal cells grown in MCDB151 showed an undifferentiated phenotype and could be serially cultured for at least 8 passages, whereas the rather differentiated cells of the fast-growing colonies in DMEM/F12 medium (1.2 mmol/L calcium) reached senescence after 3 to 4 passages.

Low calcium concentrations were not only used for clonal expansion, but, together with appropriate serum (10% FCS) and growth factor (5 ng/ml EGF and 100 ng/ml β-NGF) concentrations, also for the initial phase of subcultivation of clonally enriched cells on fibrin gels. By dissociating and transferring primary holoclones before adjacent colonies merged, the subcultured cell population became enriched with proliferative progenitor cells. Fibrin was selected as a suitable substrate, because it has been previously shown to support cell proliferation and to be

Discussion

degraded within 24 hours after transplantation [28]. However, culture conditions were switched to medium-level calcium concentrations (0.4 mmol/L) after 7 days in order to promote the development of proper cell adhesions required for establishing a multilayered epithelial cell sheet and to simultaneously allow maintainance of stem and progenitor cells within its basal layer.

This proposed culture protocol is supposed to support the survival of limbal stem and progenitor cells during the entire cultivation process, as demonstrated by immunohistochemical verification of acknowledged molecular SC markers, such as p63α, Bmi-1, ABCG2, and K15 in both holoclones and the basal layer of multilayered epithelial cell sheets. Although the presence of holoclones in cultured limbal grafts has been evaluated in one previous study [29], this is the first study to demonstrate the preservation of SC in a fibrin-based epithelial construct by using multiple molecular SC markers. Immunodetection of ΔNp63α and Bmi-1 has been previously described as an important method for identification of SC-derived holoclones and the presence of SC within a cultured graft [6, 24, 29, 30, 42, 43, 75]. Analysis of CFE of cells dissociated from the fibrin matrix indicated the persistence of SC at a percentage of 0.15% of total cell number. However, increasing the calcium concentration to 1.2mmol/L induced gradual loss of progenitor cells, as reflected by a marked decline of p63α, Bmi-1 and K15 staining and an increase in K3/K12 expression. Thus, the commonly applied culture methods using high calcium concentrations and air lifting, do not support preservation of SC, but promote terminal differentiation of TAC. However, the proposed submersion culture system using low- to medium-level calcium concentrations, appropriate serum concentrations and growth factor combinations, can be used to reconstitute transplantable cohesive sheets of partly differentiated epithelial cells retaining undifferentiated stem and progenitor cells in their basal layer.

In conclusion, we propose an improved culture protocol using biopsies from the superior limbus, a gentle two-step enzymatic dissociation method, clonal expansion of isolated SC followed by subcultivation of holoclones on fibrin in a defined environment supporting the preservation of stem and progenitor cells during the culture process. Whether this culture technique in fact enhances the therapeutic potential of limbal SC transplantation still remains to be evaluated. Nevertheless, this culture system might represent a starting point for establishing a true SC-based therapy for long-term ocular surface reconstruction, which may be further improved for clinical use, e.g. by excluding xenobiotic products, such as FCS and 3T3 feeder cells, from the culture system [76]. Moreover, for an extended survival of SC in the cultured graft, factors reproducing several aspects of the niche environment have to be integrated into the culture system in future.

5.2. Alternative sources of adult epithelial stem cells: transdifferentiation of murine and human hair follicle

Reconstruction of the stratified ocular surface epithelium in patients with bilateral LSCD is one of the most challenging problems in clinical ophthalmology. In order to replenish the SC pool, it is clearly desirable to use autologous cells for *ex vivo* culture, tissue engineering and transplantation, as this avoids the risk of allogenic immune rejection and the need for immunosuppression. A major strategy is based on autologous SC taken from stratified epithelia of other areas of the body. Recent progress in this field suggests that oral mucosal epithelium [33-35], conjunctival epithelium [36, 37], and epidermis [77, 78] may serve as alternative sources of autologous adult SC, which can be used to reconstruct the ocular surface in animal models and patients with LSCD. However, insufficient clinical long-term outcomes justify a continued search for new autologous SC sources.

The HF and its connective tissue sheath contain several, not yet completely defined SC populations with multipotent capacities [79]. Mesenchymal and nestin-expressing cells in the HF bulge region have been shown to be able to differentiate into neuronal, glial, smooth muscle, adipocytic, melanocytic, and other phenotypes in vitro [80-82]. In addition, the HF represents a major repository of multipotent keratinocyte SC in both mouse and human skin, which have the potential to differentiate into HF, sebaceous gland, and epidermis [83]. It has been even suggested that the HF bulge area contains the ultimate SC of the entire epidermis/HF compartment [48, 84, 85]. The potential of HF SC to differentiate into corneal epithelial cells has, however, not been investigated so far.

A comparison of the corneal epithelium and the follicular epithelium reveals that keratinocyte SC of these two systems share several features, such as expression of K15, K19, p63, α6 integrin, and ß1 integrin [84]. Both SC populations reside in special microenvironments involving the basement membrane components type IV collagen and laminin-5 [9] as well as close spatial association with neighbouring mesenchymal cells. Consistently, it has been demonstrated that corneal epithelium can be re-programmed to form epidermis and HF by dermal developmental signals in tissue recombination experiments [86, 87]. These observations provided the rationale for the present study presuming that HF epithelial SC might in turn be able to transdifferentiate into a corneal epithelial phenotype in response to corneal- or limbus-specific microenvironmental conditions. These microenvironmental conditions have been partially replicated *in vitro* using characteristic extracellular matrix components and fibroblast conditioned media (CM) containing specific soluble factors and signalling molecules.

The findings of the present study confirmed that holoclone forming adult SC are clustered in the bulge region of either murine vibrissae or human scalp HF [88-90] and that bulge SC can be effectively isolated both by mechanical dissection/enzymatic dissociation and fluorescence-activated cell sorting using α6 integrin labeling. The findings provided first-time evidence that epithelial HF SC can transdifferentiate into a corneal epithelial-like cell lineage after clonal

Discussion

enrichment on a feeder layer and subcultivation under conditions mimicking the limbal rather than the corneal microenvironment. In response to elevated extracellular calcium concentration and limbal fibroblast CM, both murine and human HF keratinocytes expressed significantly higher mRNA and protein levels of K12, a marker of terminally differentiated corneal epithelium, as compared with CM derived from corneal fibroblast, or 3T3 fibroblasts, or unconditioned medium. In contrast, expression of K10, a marker of terminally differentiated epidermal keratinocytes, was significantly downregulated by limbal fibroblast CM as compared with the other CM, or unconditioned control. Upregulation of K12 by limbal CM was paralleled by an induction of Pax6 mRNA and protein. The paired box gene 6 (Pax6), which is the universal master control gene for eye morphogenesis, is postnatally expressed in the corneal epithelium, where it maintains the normal epithelial phenotype and acts as a transcription factor for K12 gene expression [91, 92]. The concomitant induction of K12 and Pax6 by limbal CM provides conclusive evidence of a transdifferentiation potential of HF SC into a corneal epithelial phenotype. The stratified cell sheets cultivated in limbal CM displayed morphological characteristics of corneal epithelial cells and structural integrity as indicated by the presence of desmosomes and hemidesmosomes. They could be established on fibrin gels, which represent ideal carriers for future transplantation purposes of corneal epithelial-like cell sheets due to their standardized, non-infectious, biodegradable, and adhesive properties.

The present findings confirm the importance of the limbal SC niche, which normally regulates behaviour and differentiation of limbal stem and progenitor cells, for inducing transdifferentiation into a corneal epithelial-like phenotype. They also suggest that replication of niche factors *in vitro* increases the efficiency and lineage determination of SC-based cultivation methods. Previous studies using the inductive properties of niches to direct the differentiation of SC into desired epidermal and corneal epithelial lineages focussed primarily on mouse embryonic SC [93-96]. These were either co-cultivated with stromal fibroblasts [94], cultivated with specific matrix components and fibroblast-conditioned media [93, 97], or injected into an appropriate environment in animal models *in vivo* [95, 96]. Expression levels of K1/K10 and K3/K12 were used as an indication for differentiation into an epidermal or corneal epithelial lineage, respectively. These studies demonstrated that corneal epithelial-like cells can be obtained from embryonic SC, if they are given limbus-specific differentiation signals and environmental factors, such as type IV collagen and limbal fibroblast CM [97]. In consistency, epidermal SC obtained from adult Rhesus monkeys were demonstrated to transdifferentiate into corneal epithelial-like cells when co-cultured with human corneal limbal stroma and corneal epithelial cells [77].

As an extension of the *ex vivo* transdifferentiation studies, a preliminary engraftment experiment was performed as a starting point for *in vivo* functional studies in animal models. For this purpose human epithelial HF-derived fibrin-based constructs, pre-cultivated in limbal CM, were engrafted onto rabbit eyes with LSCD in order to access the clinical usability and efficacy of these transplants for ocular surface reconstruction. After transplantation of the HF construct onto the

Discussion

ocular surface of the damaged eyes the corneas showed complete epithelialization, no signs of inflammation, and stable, transparent, non-vascularized ocular surfaces after one week post engraftment. The expression of both the cornea-specific marker K12 as well as the epidermal differentiation marker K10 in the engrafted HF epithelial sheet, suggests that postoperatively the pre-conditioned HF epithelium maintains a corneal epithelial-like phenotype, while partly retaining the innate characteristics of epidermis. These preliminary observations suggest that HF-derived fibrin-based epithelial sheets allow corneal epithelial regeneration and promote ocular surface healing and may, therefore, be successfully used to treat patients with bilateral LSCD. However, to confirm our preliminary transplantation results, studies with a greater number of animals and with considerably longer follow-up examinations are required to provide more information on the long-term efficacy of this treatment modality. Furthermore, a thorough comparative study of the clinical outcomes using transplants composed of cultivated cells derived from various alternative autologous tissue sources like oral mucosa or conjunctiva [35] needs to be carried out to identify the most effective approach for corneal epithelial replacement in treatment of bilateral LSCD. The long-term objective would be the translation of the preclinical findings into clinical practice through transplantation of the HF-derived epithelial constructs on human LSCD eyes.

In conclusion, our findings provide evidence that soluble limbal niche factors, i.e. CM derived from stromal fibroblasts, can induce transdifferentiation of HF-derived adult SC into a corneal epithelial-like phenotype as indicated by upregulation of K12/Pax6 expression and cellular morphology. Although our findings need further substantiation using additional *in vivo* functional studies in animal models, they provide the first step towards the design of protocols to use human autologous HF SC for replacement of the corneal epithelium in therapeutic applications. Important parallels between mouse and human HF bulge cells validated the use of the mouse as a model before starting further investigations on human HF epithelial SC. Due to their multipotency, easy accessibility, and high proliferation rate *ex vivo*, HF represent an attractive source of autologous adult SC and a promising therapeutic tool for ocular surface reconstruction and restoration of visual function in patients with bilateral ocular surface disorders.

5.3 Conclusions

In conclusion, in this work an improved culture protocol for isolation, enrichment and preservation of limbal epithelial stem and progenitor cells within transplantable cultivated epithelial cell sheets for ocular surface reconstruction in patients with unilateral limbal SC deficiency was established. The proposed optimized culture procedure suggests targeted small biopsies from the superior limbus, a gentle two-step enzymatic dissociation method (dispaseII/trypsin-EDTA), clonal expansion of isolated SC on a 3T3 feeder cell layer followed by subcultivation of holoclones on a fibrin–carrier in a defined environment including low to medium calcium concentrations (0.03-0.4

Discussion

mmol), 10% serum and proper growth and survival factors combinations (EGF/NGF), preferentially supporting the preservation of stem and progenitor cells during the entire culture process prior to transplantation. Besides, this is the first study to prove the preservation of SC in a transplantable fibrin-based epithelial construct by using multiple molecular SC markers such as K15, p63α, ABCG-2, Notch-1 and Bmi-1. However, whether this culture technique in fact is able to advance the therapeutic potential of limbal SC transplantation in the clinical setting still remains to be evaluated. Nevertheless, this culture system might represent a basis for establishing a true SC-based therapy for long-term ocular surface reconstruction, which may be further improved for clinical use, e.g. by excluding xenobiotic products, such as serum and 3T3 feeder cells, from the culture system. Moreover, for an extended survival of SC in the cultured graft, specific growth and survival factors as well as extracellular matrix components mimicking several aspects of the limbal niche environment have to be integrated into the culture system in future.

Furthermore, the present findings provide evidence that soluble and matrix-associated specific limbal niche factors, i.e. CM derived from limbal stromal fibroblasts and laminin-5, can induce transdifferentiation of both murine and human HF-derived SC into a corneal epithelial-like phenotype as indicated by upregulation of cornea-specific marker (K12, Pax6) expression and cellular morphology. Although these findings need further substantiation using *in vivo* functional studies with a greater number of animals and various experimental animal models, they provide the first step towards tissue engineering approaches using human autologous HF SC for replacement of the corneal epithelium in therapeutic applications. Due to their multipotency, easy accessibility, and high proliferation rate *ex vivo*, HF-derived SC represent an attractive source of autologous adult SC and a promising therapeutic tool for ocular surface reconstruction and restoration of visual function in patients with ocular surface disorders.

6. References

1. Lavker RM, Sun TT. Epithelial stem cells: the eye provides a vision. *Eye.* 2003;17:937-942.

2. Cotsarelis G, Cheng SZ, Dong G, Sun TT, Lavker RM. Existence of slow-cycling limbal epithelial basal cells that can be preferentially stimulated to proliferate: implications on epithelial stem cells. *Cell.* 1989;57:201-209.

3. Schlotzer-Schrehardt U, Kruse FE. Identification and characterization of limbal stem cells. *Exp Eye Res.* 2005;81:247-264.

4. Lavker RM, Dong G, Cheng SZ et al. Relative proliferative rates of limbal and corneal epithelia. Implications of corneal epithelial migration, circadian rhythm, and suprabasally located DNA-synthesizing keratinocytes. *Invest Ophthalmol Vis Sci.* 1991;32:1864-1875.

5. Romano AC, Espana EM, Yoo SH et al. Different cell sizes in human limbal and central corneal basal epithelia measured by confocal microscopy and flow cytometry. *Invest Ophthalmol Vis Sci.* 2003;44:5125-5129.

6. Pellegrini G, Rama P, Mavilio F, De Luca M. Epithelial stem cells in corneal regeneration and epidermal gene therapy. *J Pathol.* 2009;217:217-228.

7. Davanger M, Evensen A. Role of the pericorneal papillary structure in renewal of corneal epithelium. *Nature.* 1971;229:560-561.

8. Tseng SC. Regulation and clinical implications of corneal epithelial stem cells. *Mol Biol Rep.* 1996;23:47-58.

9. Schlotzer-Schrehardt U, Dietrich T, Saito K et al. Characterization of extracellular matrix components in the limbal epithelial stem cell compartment. *Exp Eye Res.* 2007;85:845-860.

10. Li W, Hayashida Y, Chen YT, Tseng SC. Niche regulation of corneal epithelial stem cells at the limbus. *Cell Res.* 2007;17:26-36.

11. Li DQ, Tseng SC. Three patterns of cytokine expression potentially involved in epithelial-fibroblast interactions of human ocular surface. *J Cell Physiol.* 1995;163:61-79.

12. Ihanamaki T, Pelliniemi LJ, Vuorio E. Collagens and collagen-related matrix components in the human and mouse eye. *Prog Retin Eye Res.* 2004;23:403-434.

13. Erickson AC, Couchman JR. Still more complexity in mammalian basement membranes. *J Histochem Cytochem.* 2000;48:1291-1306.

References

14. Qi H, Li DQ, Shine HD et al. Nerve growth factor and its receptor TrkA serve as potential markers for human corneal epithelial progenitor cells. *Exp Eye Res.* 2008;86:34-40.

15. Qi H, Chuang EY, Yoon KC et al. Patterned expression of neurotrophic factors and receptors in human limbal and corneal regions. *Mol Vis.* 2007;13:1934-1941.

16. Klenkler BJ, Griffith M, Becerril C, West-Mays JA, Sheardown H. EGF-grafted PDMS surfaces in artificial cornea applications. *Biomaterials.* 2005;26:7286-7296.

17. Daniels JT, Dart JK, Tuft SJ, Khaw PT. Corneal stem cells in review. *Wound Repair Regen.* 2001;9:483-494.

18. Pellegrini G, Traverso CE, Franzi AT et al. Long-term restoration of damaged corneal surfaces with autologous cultivated corneal epithelium. *Lancet.* 1997;349:990-993.

19. Shortt AJ, Secker GA, Notara MD et al. Transplantation of ex vivo cultured limbal epithelial stem cells: a review of techniques and clinical results. *Surv Ophthalmol.* 2007;52:483-502.

20. Shimazaki J, Maruyama F, Shimmura S, Fujishima H, Tsubota K. Immunologic rejection of the central graft after limbal allograft transplantation combined with penetrating keratoplasty. *Cornea.* 2001;20:149-152.

21. Daya SM, Watson A, Sharpe JR et al. Outcomes and DNA analysis of ex vivo expanded stem cell allograft for ocular surface reconstruction. *Ophthalmology.* 2005;112:470-477.

22. Sharpe JR, Daya SM, Dimitriadi M, Martin R, James SE. Survival of cultured allogeneic limbal epithelial cells following corneal repair. *Tissue Eng.* 2007;13:123-132.

23. Li W, Hayashida Y, He H, Kuo CL, Tseng SC. The fate of limbal epithelial progenitor cells during explant culture on intact amniotic membrane. *Invest Ophthalmol Vis Sci.* 2007;48:605-613.

24. Pellegrini G, De Luca M, Arsenijevic Y. Towards therapeutic application of ocular stem cells. *Semin Cell Dev Biol.* 2007;18:805-818.

25. Rheinwald JG, Green H. Serial cultivation of strains of human epidermal keratinocytes: the formation of keratinizing colonies from single cells. *Cell.* 1975;6:331-343.

26. Tseng SC, Kruse FE, Merritt J, Li DQ. Comparison between serum-free and fibroblast-cocultured single-cell clonal culture systems: evidence showing that epithelial anti-apoptotic activity is present in 3T3 fibroblast-conditioned media. *Curr Eye Res.* 1996;15:973-984.

References

27. Barrandon Y, Green H. Three clonal types of keratinocyte with different capacities for multiplication. *Proc Natl Acad Sci U S A.* 1987;84:2302-2306.

28. Pellegrini G, Ranno R, Stracuzzi G et al. The control of epidermal stem cells (holoclones) in the treatment of massive full-thickness burns with autologous keratinocytes cultured on fibrin. *Transplantation.* 1999;68:868-879.

29. Rama P, Bonini S, Lambiase A et al. Autologous fibrin-cultured limbal stem cells permanently restore the corneal surface of patients with total limbal stem cell deficiency. *Transplantation.* 2001;72:1478-1485.

30. De Luca M, Pellegrini G, Green H. Regeneration of squamous epithelia from stem cells of cultured grafts. *Regen Med.* 2006;1:45-57.

31. Ronfard V, Rives JM, Neveux Y, Carsin H, Barrandon Y. Long-term regeneration of human epidermis on third degree burns transplanted with autologous cultured epithelium grown on a fibrin matrix. *Transplantation.* 2000;70:1588-1598.

32. Mavilio F, Pellegrini G, Ferrari S et al. Correction of junctional epidermolysis bullosa by transplantation of genetically modified epidermal stem cells. *Nat Med.* 2006;12:1397-1402.

33. Nakamura T, Kinoshita S. Ocular surface reconstruction using cultivated mucosal epithelial stem cells. *Cornea.* 2003;22:S75-80.

34. Nishida K, Yamato M, Hayashida Y et al. Corneal reconstruction with tissue-engineered cell sheets composed of autologous oral mucosal epithelium. *N Engl J Med.* 2004;351:1187-1196.

35. Inatomi T, Nakamura T, Koizumi N et al. Midterm results on ocular surface reconstruction using cultivated autologous oral mucosal epithelial transplantation. *Am J Ophthalmol.* 2006;141:267-275.

36. Tanioka H, Kawasaki S, Yamasaki K et al. Establishment of a cultivated human conjunctival epithelium as an alternative tissue source for autologous corneal epithelial transplantation. *Invest Ophthalmol Vis Sci.* 2006;47:3820-3827.

37. Ono K, Yokoo S, Mimura T et al. Autologous transplantation of conjunctival epithelial cells cultured on amniotic membrane in a rabbit model. *Mol Vis.* 2007;13:1138-1143.

38. Yano S, Okochi H. Long-term culture of adult murine epidermal keratinocytes. *Br J Dermatol.* 2005;153:1101-1104.

References

39. Zenkel M, Kruse FE, Naumann GO, Schlotzer-Schrehardt U. Impaired cytoprotective mechanisms in eyes with pseudoexfoliation syndrome/glaucoma. *Invest Ophthalmol Vis Sci.* 2007;48:5558-5566.

40. Jones PH, Watt FM. Separation of human epidermal stem cells from transit amplifying cells on the basis of differences in integrin function and expression. *Cell.* 1993;73:713-724.

41. Pellegrini G, Golisano O, Paterna P et al. Location and clonal analysis of stem cells and their differentiated progeny in the human ocular surface. *J Cell Biol.* 1999;145:769-782.

42. Di Iorio E, Barbaro V, Ruzza A et al. Isoforms of DeltaNp63 and the migration of ocular limbal cells in human corneal regeneration. *Proc Natl Acad Sci U S A.* 2005;102:9523-9528.

43. Di Iorio E, Barbaro V, Ferrari S et al. Q-FIHC: quantification of fluorescence immunohistochemistry to analyse p63 isoforms and cell cycle phases in human limbal stem cells. *Microsc Res Tech.* 2006;69:983-991.

44. Kruse FE, Tseng SC. Proliferative and differentiative response of corneal and limbal epithelium to extracellular calcium in serum-free clonal cultures. *J Cell Physiol.* 1992;151:347-360.

45. Barnard Z, Apel AJ, Harkin DG. Phenotypic analyses of limbal epithelial cell cultures derived from donor corneoscleral rims. *Clin Experiment Ophthalmol.* 2001;29:138-142.

46. Lavker RM, Sun TT. Epidermal stem cells: properties, markers, and location. *Proc Natl Acad Sci U S A.* 2000;97:13473-13475.

47. Jensen UB, Yan X, Triel C et al. A distinct population of clonogenic and multipotent murine follicular keratinocytes residing in the upper isthmus. *J Cell Sci.* 2008;121:609-617.

48. Blanpain C, Lowry WE, Geoghegan A, Polak L, Fuchs E. Self-renewal, multipotency, and the existence of two cell populations within an epithelial stem cell niche. *Cell.* 2004;118:635-648.

49. Tsai RJ, Li LM, Chen JK. Reconstruction of damaged corneas by transplantation of autologous limbal epithelial cells. *N Engl J Med.* 2000;343:86-93.

50. Koizumi N, Inatomi T, Suzuki T, Sotozono C, Kinoshita S. Cultivated corneal epithelial stem cell transplantation in ocular surface disorders. *Ophthalmology.* 2001;108:1569-1574.

References

51. Shimazaki J, Aiba M, Goto E et al. Transplantation of human limbal epithelium cultivated on amniotic membrane for the treatment of severe ocular surface disorders. *Ophthalmology.* 2002;109:1285-1290.

52. Grueterich M, Espana EM, Touhami A, Ti SE, Tseng SC. Phenotypic study of a case with successful transplantation of ex vivo expanded human limbal epithelium for unilateral total limbal stem cell deficiency. *Ophthalmology.* 2002;109:1547-1552.

53. Sangwan VS, Vemuganti GK, Singh S, Balasubramanian D. Successful reconstruction of damaged ocular outer surface in humans using limbal and conjuctival stem cell culture methods. *Biosci Rep.* 2003;23:169-174.

54. Nakamura T, Inatomi T, Sotozono C, Koizumi N, Kinoshita S. Successful primary culture and autologous transplantation of corneal limbal epithelial cells from minimal biopsy for unilateral severe ocular surface disease. *Acta Ophthalmol Scand.* 2004;82:468-471.

55. Schwab IR, Reyes M, Isseroff RR. Successful transplantation of bioengineered tissue replacements in patients with ocular surface disease. *Cornea.* 2000;19:421-426.

56. Koizumi N, Cooper LJ, Fullwood NJ et al. An evaluation of cultivated corneal limbal epithelial cells, using cell-suspension culture. *Invest Ophthalmol Vis Sci.* 2002;43:2114-2121.

57. Kim HS, Jun Song X, de Paiva CS et al. Phenotypic characterization of human corneal epithelial cells expanded ex vivo from limbal explant and single cell cultures. *Exp Eye Res.* 2004;79:41-49.

58. Zhang X, Sun H, Tang X et al. Comparison of cell-suspension and explant culture of rabbit limbal epithelial cells. *Exp Eye Res.* 2005;80:227-233.

59. Nakamura T, Inatomi T, Sotozono C et al. Transplantation of autologous serum-derived cultivated corneal epithelial equivalents for the treatment of severe ocular surface disease. *Ophthalmology.* 2006;113:1765-1772.

60. Barrandon Y. Crossing boundaries: stem cells, holoclones, and the fundamentals of squamous epithelial renewal. *Cornea.* 2007;26:S10-12.

61. Shimmura S, Tsubota K. Surgical treatment of limbal stem cell deficiency: are we really transplanting stem cells? *Am J Ophthalmol.* 2008;146:154-155.

62. Lauweryns B, van den Oord JJ, De Vos R, Missotten L. A new epithelial cell type in the human cornea. *Invest Ophthalmol Vis Sci.* 1993;34:1983-1990.

References

63. Wiley L, SundarRaj N, Sun TT, Thoft RA. Regional heterogeneity in human corneal and limbal epithelia: an immunohistochemical evaluation. *Invest Ophthalmol Vis Sci.* 1991;32:594-602.

64. Shortt AJ, Secker GA, Munro PM et al. Characterization of the limbal epithelial stem cell niche: novel imaging techniques permit in vivo observation and targeted biopsy of limbal epithelial stem cells. *Stem Cells.* 2007;25:1402-1409.

65. Kruse FE, Tseng SC. Serum differentially modulates the clonal growth and differentiation of cultured limbal and corneal epithelium. *Invest Ophthalmol Vis Sci.* 1993;34:2976-2989.

66. Kruse FE, Tseng SC. Retinoic acid regulates clonal growth and differentiation of cultured limbal and peripheral corneal epithelium. *Invest Ophthalmol Vis Sci.* 1994;35:2405-2420.

67. Rheinwald JG, Green H. Epidermal growth factor and the multiplication of cultured human epidermal keratinocytes. *Nature.* 1977;265:421-424.

68. Sun TT, Green H. Cultured epithelial cells of cornea, conjunctiva and skin: absence of marked intrinsic divergence of their differentiated states. *Nature.* 1977;269:489-493.

69. Li DQ, Tseng SC. Differential regulation of keratinocyte growth factor and hepatocyte growth factor/scatter factor by different cytokines in human corneal and limbal fibroblasts. *J Cell Physiol.* 1997;172:361-372.

70. Lambiase A, Rama P, Bonini S, Caprioglio G, Aloe L. Topical treatment with nerve growth factor for corneal neurotrophic ulcers. *N Engl J Med.* 1998;338:1174-1180.

71. Touhami A, Grueterich M, Tseng SC. The role of NGF signaling in human limbal epithelium expanded by amniotic membrane culture. *Invest Ophthalmol Vis Sci.* 2002;43:987-994.

72. Hennings H, Michael D, Cheng C et al. Calcium regulation of growth and differentiation of mouse epidermal cells in culture. *Cell.* 1980;19:245-254.

73. Kawakita T, Espana EM, He H et al. Calcium-induced abnormal epidermal-like differentiation in cultures of mouse corneal-limbal epithelial cells. *Invest Ophthalmol Vis Sci.* 2004;45:3507-3512.

74. Kawakita T, Shimmura S, Hornia A, Higa K, Tseng SC. Stratified epithelial sheets engineered from a single adult murine corneal/limbal progenitor cell. *J Cell Mol Med.* 2008.

75. Barbaro V, Testa A, Di Iorio E et al. C/EBPdelta regulates cell cycle and self-renewal of human limbal stem cells. *J Cell Biol.* 2007;177:1037-1049.

References

76. Omoto M, Miyashita H, Shimmura S et al. The use of human mesenchymal stem cell-derived feeder cells for the cultivation of transplantable epithelial sheets. *Invest Ophthalmol Vis Sci.* 2009.

77. Gao N, Wang Z, Huang B et al. Putative epidermal stem cell convert into corneal epithelium-like cell under corneal tissue in vitro. *Sci China C Life Sci.* 2007;50:101-110.

78. Yang X, Qu L, Wang X et al. Plasticity of epidermal adult stem cells derived from adult goat ear skin. *Mol Reprod Dev.* 2007;74:386-396.

79. Tiede S, Kloepper JE, Bodo E et al. Hair follicle stem cells: walking the maze. *Eur J Cell Biol.* 2007;86:355-376.

80. Amoh Y, Li L, Katsuoka K, Hoffman RM. Multipotent hair follicle stem cells promote repair of spinal cord injury and recovery of walking function. *Cell Cycle.* 2008;7.

81. Mignone JL, Roig-Lopez JL, Fedtsova N et al. Neural potential of a stem cell population in the hair follicle. *Cell Cycle.* 2007;6:2161-2170.

82. Hoffman RM. The potential of nestin-expressing hair follicle stem cells in regenerative medicine. *Expert Opin Biol Ther.* 2007;7:289-291.

83. Ito M, Liu Y, Yang Z et al. Stem cells in the hair follicle bulge contribute to wound repair but not to homeostasis of the epidermis. *Nat Med.* 2005;11:1351-1354.

84. Taylor G, Lehrer MS, Jensen PJ, Sun TT, Lavker RM. Involvement of follicular stem cells in forming not only the follicle but also the epidermis. *Cell.* 2000;102:451-461.

85. Levy V, Lindon C, Zheng Y, Harfe BD, Morgan BA. Epidermal stem cells arise from the hair follicle after wounding. *FASEB J.* 2007;21:1358-1366.

86. Ferraris C, Chevalier G, Favier B, Jahoda CA, Dhouailly D. Adult corneal epithelium basal cells possess the capacity to activate epidermal, pilosebaceous and sweat gland genetic programs in response to embryonic dermal stimuli. *Development.* 2000;127:5487-5495.

87. Pearton DJ, Ferraris C, Dhouailly D. Transdifferentiation of corneal epithelium: evidence for a linkage between the segregation of epidermal stem cells and the induction of hair follicles during embryogenesis. *Int J Dev Biol.* 2004;48:197-201.

88. Lavker RM, Sun TT, Oshima H et al. Hair follicle stem cells. *J Investig Dermatol Symp Proc.* 2003;8:28-38.

References

89. Morris RJ, Liu Y, Marles L et al. Capturing and profiling adult hair follicle stem cells. *Nat Biotechnol.* 2004;22:411-417.

90. Ohyama M. Hair follicle bulge: a fascinating reservoir of epithelial stem cells. *J Dermatol Sci.* 2007;46:81-89.

91. Shiraishi A, Converse RL, Liu CY et al. Identification of the cornea-specific keratin 12 promoter by in vivo particle-mediated gene transfer. *Invest Ophthalmol Vis Sci.* 1998;39:2554-2561.

92. Li W, Chen YT, Hayashida Y et al. Down-regulation of Pax6 is associated with abnormal differentiation of corneal epithelial cells in severe ocular surface diseases. *J Pathol.* 2008;214:114-122.

93. Homma R, Yoshikawa H, Takeno M et al. Induction of epithelial progenitors in vitro from mouse embryonic stem cells and application for reconstruction of damaged cornea in mice. *Invest Ophthalmol Vis Sci.* 2004;45:4320-4326.

94. Coraux C, Hilmi C, Rouleau M et al. Reconstituted skin from murine embryonic stem cells. *Curr Biol.* 2003;13:849-853.

95. Bagutti C, Wobus AM, Fassler R, Watt FM. Differentiation of embryonal stem cells into keratinocytes: comparison of wild-type and beta 1 integrin-deficient cells. *Dev Biol.* 1996;179:184-196.

96. Green H, Easley K, Iuchi S. Marker succession during the development of keratinocytes from cultured human embryonic stem cells. *Proc Natl Acad Sci U S A.* 2003;100:15625-15630.

97. Ahmad S, Stewart R, Yung S et al. Differentiation of human embryonic stem cells into corneal epithelial-like cells by in vitro replication of the corneal epithelial stem cell niche. *Stem Cells.* 2007;25:1145-1155.

7. Abbreviations

BDNF: brain-derived neurotrophic factor
BM: basement membrane
ß-NGF: nerve growth factor
Ca: calcium
$CaCl_2$: calcium chloride
cDNA: copy desoxyribonucleic acid
CFE: colony-forming efficiency
cm: cenimeter
DAPI: 4´,6´-diamino-2-phenylindole
D-KSFM: Defined Keratinocyte Serum-Free medium
DMEM/F12: Dulbecco´s modified Eagle´s medium and Ham´s F12 medium
DOC: Deoxycholate
EDTA: ethylenediaminetetraaceticacid
EGF: epidermal growth factor
e.g.: for example
FACS: fluorescence activated cell sorting
FCS: fetal calf serum
FGF: basic fibroblast growth factor
GDNF: glial cell-derived neurotrophic factor
HCGS: human corneal growth supplement
HCl: hydrochloric acid
HF: hair follicle
HGF: hepatocyte growth factor
IGF-I: insulin-like growth factor-I
kDa: kilodalton
KGF: keratinocyte growth factor
LIF: leukemia inhibitory factor
LSCD: limbal stem cell deficiency
$MgCl_2$: magnesium chloride
min: minute
ml: millilitre
mM: millimolar
µm: micrometer
NaCl: natrium chloride
PAGE: polyacrylamide gel electrophoresis

Abbreviations

PBS: phosphate-buffered saline
PCT medium: Progenitor Cell Targeting medium
PDGF-BB: platelet-derived growth factor-BB
RIPA: radioimmunoprecipitation
SC: stem cell(s)
SCF: stem cell factor
SDS: sodium dodecyle sulphate
sec: second
TGF-α: transforming growth factor-α
U: unit

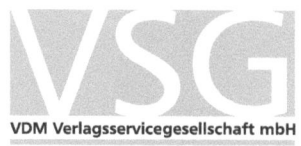

Die VDM Verlagsservicegesellschaft sucht für wissenschaftliche Verlage abgeschlossene und herausragende

Dissertationen, Habilitationen, Diplomarbeiten, Master Theses, Magisterarbeiten usw.

für die kostenlose Publikation als Fachbuch.

Sie verfügen über eine Arbeit, die hohen inhaltlichen und formalen Ansprüchen genügt, und haben Interesse an einer honorarvergüteten Publikation?

Dann senden Sie bitte erste Informationen über sich und Ihre Arbeit per Email an *info@vdm-vsg.de*.

Sie erhalten kurzfristig unser Feedback!

VDM Verlagsservicegesellschaft mbH
Dudweiler Landstr. 99   Telefon +49 681 3720 174
D - 66123 Saarbrücken   Fax   +49 681 3720 1749
www.vdm-vsg.de

Die VDM Verlagsservicegesellschaft mbH vertritt

 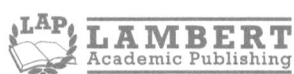 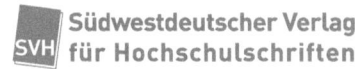

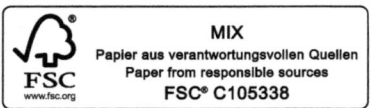

Printed by Books on Demand GmbH, Norderstedt / Germany